Lose Weight
And Be Healthy Now

Forty Science-Based
Weight Loss Tips
To Transform Your Life

David Bennett
and Jonathan Bennett

Amazing Cover Design: Ashley Ware
www.artofaware.com

Internal Photographs: David Bennett

Theta Hill Press

Lancaster, Ohio

thetahillpress.com

Theta Hill Press

Copyright © 2015 Theta Hill Press

ISBN: 0692543937

ISBN-13: 978-0692543931

Medical Disclaimer

Information in this book is intended as an educational aid only. No information contained in this book should be construed as medical or psychological advice, diagnosis, or treatment. The material in this book should not be taken as the advice of a physician or dietician. Readers should consult appropriate health professionals on any matter relating to their health and well-being, and before starting any diet, exercise, or health improvement regimen, and follow the advice of those professionals.

TABLE OF CONTENTS

SOME GROUND RULES

Remember everyone. This book should NOT be construed as medical advice or the advice of a dietician. This is for informational purposes only, and is akin to reading what a journalist or blogger has to say about weight loss. Consult a healthcare professional before undertaking any weight loss, exercise, or health improvement process.

This book isn't about easy answers, quick fixes, or expensive fads. I would say Jonathan and I have "tried it all," but the truth is we haven't tried a lot of the expensive junk. The weight loss industry is out to make money. I have no problem with that…that's why it's called an "industry." However, that doesn't mean most of the products or programs work, or that we are going to peddle anything like that here.

Jonathan and my weight loss journey, where a lot of the tips in this book come from, took us on the opposite path: finding scientifically grounded tips that could give us an advantage when shedding pounds. In other words, we started learning the simple and cheap stuff that works! And, we are going to share that with you here.

The tips in this book presuppose a few things, so take note:

- This book is not a diet book! While we adhere to a lower calorie and lower carb diet philosophy (I usually get anywhere from 1700-2300 calories a day and try to keep my carbs in the 75-175 range), and enjoy meat, other diet plans work to lose weight as well.

If you are trying to lose weight, find a program that works well for you. Low carb works for me because not only does it deliver results, but I can eat the foods I like. It also makes me feel emotionally and physically energetic.

- This book is not going to give you a list of exercises. I assume you are exercising and learning about ways to do it, whether you are taking up running, playing a sport, or using an at home program like Insanity.

- Losing weight requires effort. There is no "quick fix" or miracle pill. If a miracle pill existed to make you lose weight fast we would probably call it what it is: a poison! That is what we call chemicals that cause quick weight loss.

- While it is important to love yourself, no matter how unhealthy, overweight, or out-of-shape you are, getting healthy is the best way to become your best self. If you are overweight, you will look and feel better if you shed the excess pounds, and we assume you are reading this as a motivated person, ready to get to work! There is no shaming in this book (shame doesn't work), but we do want to empower you!

- If you have been diagnosed with an eating disorder, or your loved ones suggest that you have one, get help. This book is not for you. Seriously. Seek proper help and don't read this book.

- Some of these tips may seem like "common sense." I'm sure someone will level that complaint. However, that still doesn't mean most readers are actually following common sense advice. If a few of the chapters remind you of the common sense stuff you should be doing, then this book is giving you value!

- This book references many smaller scientific studies. I am aware that research carried out over a longer duration with bigger sample sizes could end up disproving some of these tips.

Since the tips here are cheap, easy to do, and may have other benefits besides weight loss, trying them out won't hurt you even if they are later disproven by larger studies. We have attempted to link to the various sources throughout the book.

- Since I am writing this with my brother Jonathan, the author of each tip is indicated at the end of the chapter. That will help you keep our stories and anecdotes straight.

Okay...without further ado, here is my story!

- David

DAVID'S STORY

I have struggled to lose weight since middle school. In middle school I discovered the wonders of video games, cafeteria food, and a huge breakfast. My life pretty much revolved around delicious food. I woke up to the smell of my dad pan frying sausage, and by the time I was fully awake, I was chomping down two huge sausage sandwiches.

For lunch, I had a mini pizza, a pack of peanuts, and a "honey bun" doughnut. Dinner depended on the day, but I loved when our family dined out on Friday nights. At the local burger joint "Sumburger," my order was consistent: two plain cheeseburgers, deep fried mushrooms, and a large Pepsi.

My estimate of the calories from an average day like that is about 2700. If I were working hard at football practice, or playing pick-up basketball all day with my friends, then that wouldn't be a huge deal. Actually, I was playing a lot of football and basketball…on the Nintendo. I loved Tecmo Bowl and Double Dribble.

In fifth grade, I had a chance to take a special overnight field trip for gifted kids. We got to tour the Ohio River area, and even ride on (and steer) a real steamboat! When I saw the itinerary beforehand my only concern was the food. While other kids were probably concerned about having fun and seeing their friends, I was mapping out in my head when my meals would come.

In seventh grade, my school offered a class called "Weighty Matters." At that age, I didn't get the pun, but I did attend a few sessions, because I knew I needed to lose a little weight. I remember two things from that class. First, the nurse smeared margarine on a bun to show how much fat was in a Big Mac. Second, she passed out a document with nutritional information for different foods. Upon seeing that fish was very low in calories and fat, I requested we go out to Long John Silvers for some fried fish, fries, hush puppies, and soda. So, yeah, I pretty much missed the point.

In eighth grade, my obsession with food continued. As I was preparing for a band trip to sunny Florida, where I would visit beaches and a major theme park, all I was worried about was food. I packed thirty packets of candy for the trip, to make sure I was well-nourished. While other kids were worried about socializing and getting a tan on the beach, I was counting the food items to be sure I really did get a seven course meal at the medieval themed restaurant. I did learn that a can of Coke counts as a "course" and I wasn't too happy about that.

Ironically, it was that same week that my dad, in his early forties, had a mini-stroke. He had been obese for years, and it was taking its toll. He woke up one morning and couldn't remember anything. He eventually recovered his memories, and functions perfectly now, but it was a wake-up call for our family.

Suddenly, we were eating ground turkey instead of beef, and Diet Rite instead of Coke. Our family decided it was time to get healthy. We all benefited from the changes. My dad did end up losing about eighty pounds (sadly, he gained it back). That finally got me seriously thinking about health.

When I was a freshman in high school I finally got the "health vision." I reached a point where I was sick of being out of shape and unpopular. I basically reinvented myself. My brother checked *Lendon Smith's Diet Plan For Teenagers* out of the library and that sparked my interest in eating right, exercising, and taking supplements.

I felt a lot better and started branching out socially. I decided I would play football my sophomore year, so I started lifting with the team the winter of my freshman year. I wish I could say my weight loss journey ended there, but it didn't, although it did get a good start.

My weight fluctuated in high school quite a bit, usually going from about 170 pounds up as high as 185. For my 5'7" frame, at 170 I looked pretty good, especially since I had a lot of muscle mass.

My weight largely fluctuated because I loved food – and lots of it. I would play softball and "go off" my diet and eat two ham and cheese subs with French fries. The lowest I ever got in high school was 167 pounds, and that was after training for a 200 mile round trip bicycle ride, along with a summer of running nearly every day and lifting weights nearly four times a week.

By the time the summer was over, I was up to running six miles. It was difficult to keep the weight off during football season. My day lasted from 7:00 AM until 7:30 PM, I was tired and stressed, and I ate to compensate. I graduated from high school heavier than I would have liked.

My weight fluctuated in college too. I went into college a little overweight, but gained more my freshman year, since I spent a lot of my time playing trivia at a local restaurant. I ate plenty of chicken wings and hamburgers that year, and didn't get much activity. The summer before my sophomore year I once again lost the weight, got a girlfriend, got lazy, and gained it back again, only to lose it again the summer going into my junior year. And, of course, I gained that back by the time I started my senior year!

Do you see a trend here? My weight fluctuated a lot when I was in high school and college.

I was at my absolute highest my senior year in college. I'm going to focus on this for a while because it was my highest and weight and the habits that led to it were disastrous.

My senior year I met my girlfriend for breakfast every morning. We decided it was something fun to do. And, if breakfast was cute, so was lunch and dinner. I started to revolve my life around food again. For breakfast I would have eggs and sausage. Lunch was a sandwich and chips, and then dinner was whatever the dining hall served – and lots of it.

What I really remember well are the late night snacks. About three nights a week, on top of what I was eating during the day, I would walk next door to the local convenience store. I bought two small bags of Doritos, washing them down with a container of whole milk. The total calorie load from my nighttime snacking was about 1000.

I ballooned to 200 pounds my senior year. My clothes didn't fit. I could hardly walk up the stairs of my dorm without getting winded, and I barely recognized myself in the mirror. For the first time ever, I had to buy pants with a waist of 37. It was a shock when I was forced to admit that I was that big.

The spring of my senior year, right before graduation, I realized something had to give.

I started eating right and going to the exercise center. It was extremely difficult. I hadn't run or worked out in a year. Spending even a few minutes on the exercise bike killed me. Nonetheless, I worked hard. I exercised regularly for about two months and nothing seemed to happen. I plateaued. My weight was basically stuck at about 195 pounds for what seemed like months.

I determined I wouldn't get discouraged. I hadn't lived in a healthy way for years. After I graduated, I took a job working at a drug and alcohol treatment center. I packed my lunch most days and avoided the donuts the other employees always brought in. I continued to run, enjoying my daily runs up and down the beautiful hills near my hometown.

By the time I went to grad school I was down to 185. Nonetheless, I was still pretty far from where I wanted to be. So, I continued working hard at grad school. My brother and I roomed together, so we would make sure we cooked healthy meals. I remember eating a lot of whole grains, ground turkey tacos, and tofu. I continued losing weight until I eventually got down to 150, virtually the lowest I have ever weighed.

We also made a conscious choice to walk from our apartment complex to our classes each day. While most of our fellow students were taking the university transport system, we chose to walk the half mile trip each morning. It was a great way to start the day, and since this was in Georgia, there was rarely a day the weather was too bad to make it happen.

I kept in a healthy weight range from grad school (2000) until around 2006. It was then that I decided that eating chicken wings four times a week while playing trivia at a local restaurant was a great idea. I became busy as a teacher and my weight ballooned again, this time back up to 195.

I couldn't believe it! I allowed myself to get back to the weight I was when I felt and looked horribly. This time I decided I couldn't let it happen again and I started keeping track of my food and exercise intake regularly with a program called "Fitday."

At first I was inconsistent. I did it in the winter of 2006, but not after. I was determined to lose weight for my wedding, so I went from 195 in late 2006 to 170 by September of 2007. The first photo at the end of the chapter is from my heavy period in the spring of 2007.

Since November 2007 I have regularly, without fail, recorded everything I have eaten, and all activity, in Fitday. It has been a very effective help in keeping me at a healthy weight. Since 2007 I have kept my weight in a healthy range. Right now I am a muscular 155.

Around 2009 I decided to write and compile some of the tips I collected over the years. These tips were originally posted on lifeinyouryears.net. This book is a collection of these tips, with plenty of updates and additions.

The reason Jonathan and I are telling our weight loss journeys is to give you some perspective. Losing weight is about living a healthy lifestyle. Eating right, exercising, and living a balanced life will make you feel amazing. You'll have more energy and look and feel younger. You'll start to get more attention from people. There are many benefits.

It is also hard at times. I'm a teacher and both students and teachers joke about my eating habits. They ask "eating more kale today?" or "is that really low carb, Mr. Bennett?" All my students have taste-tested my stevia powder.

They gently poke fun at my eating habits, but they also respect them, because they see the benefits of my lifestyle choices. I am nearly forty and just ran my fourth "Tough Mudder" race. I run after school most days, and I can mentally and physically keep up with people half my age. I often get mistaken for being in my mid to late twenties. The other day a student argued with me about my age, insisting there was no way I was 37.

My life is much richer and fuller thanks to healthy choices. There is nothing fulfilling or fun about being physically unable to fully participate in life's activities because of obesity. In fact, being healthy is an essential component of my business. Let me explain.

As the co-owner of <u>The Popular Man</u> (thepopularman.com) and <u>The Popular Teen</u> (thepopularteen.com), and author of various books designed to help men and teens develop social skills to become confident and charismatic leaders, I know the importance of looking your best.

Whether it is fair or not, attractive people are often judged as having great personalities, and they tend to get perks and benefits simply based on their looks, which is called The Halo Effect (1). This isn't right, but it is reality.

Also, studies show that the better a person's immune system, the more attractive they are to the opposite sex. For men, the more fit they are, the higher their testosterone levels, which makes guys more attractive (2). Women derive many of the same social benefits from being fit and at a healthy weight. These are just a few of the reasons why weight loss and good health are key components of our social transformation programs.

I wish you the best as you start or continue your weight loss journey. Remember that **you can do it**! The second photo at the end of this chapter is me in 2015.

- David

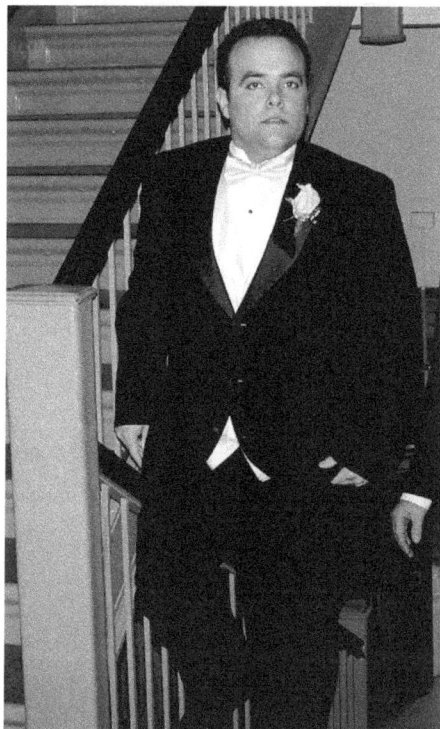

David in 2007

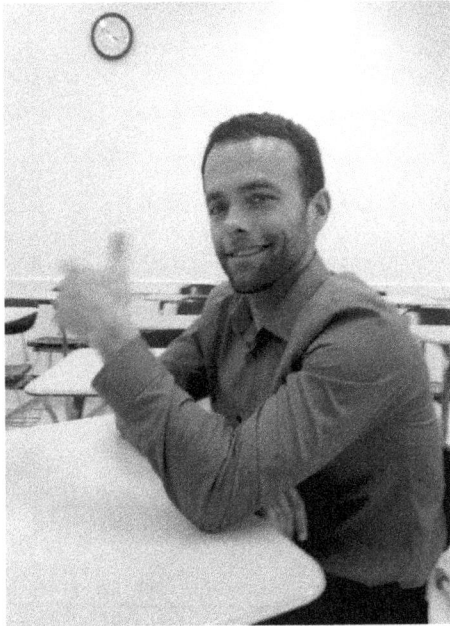

David in 2015

JONATHAN'S STORY

When I was young, I loved doing outdoor activities. You could find me swimming, playing kickball, going on hikes with the cub scouts, riding my bike down the streets and more. I was a very creative and active child. In fact, every Sunday after church it was a ritual for all the kids to play kickball.

Not only did I play kickball, but my brother and I (along with one friend) took on everybody else who wanted to play. It was literally the three of us sometimes playing ten to fifteen kids. We were legends, at least in our own minds.

However, in third grade, something changed. The Nintendo Entertainment System was released. Instead of going outside, my friends and I would go inside and play that. My active life ceased and I started to get a lot more sedentary.

This also coincided with different eating habits. When I was active, eating was an afterthought. I ate when I was hungry. However, now that I spent all my time in front of the Nintendo, it became a lot easier to go to the fridge or cabinet and eat junk food. As a result, I fell in love with food.

By age ten, I had gone from thin to fat. I was never grossly obese, but definitely fat enough that it impacted my health and self-esteem. Lunch was my favorite time of the day. I was friends with the cafeteria cooks, but otherwise sometimes ate alone. All I needed was food to be happy.

I would start the day with two sausage sandwiches, and for lunch I would often combine foods, enjoying personal pepperoni pizzas, "honey buns," peanuts, and whatever else was on the menu for that day. Dinner was often just as bad.

I stopped caring about my appearance and didn't do anything except play video games in my house. I literally wore sweat pants every day to school. Even though my grades were good, I was a mess inside and out.

In ninth grade, I finally got sick of the misery and looked for a way out. I checked out a weight loss book for teens from the library. And, I followed it. This coincided roughly with my dad having a stroke and needing to lose weight himself. My family suddenly replaced "sloppy joe night" with "turkey burger night."

That year I changed my life. I joined the football team, started lifting weights, and felt a lot like a new person. I started choosing foods on the basis of their nutritional content instead of only on how they tasted.

I ate salads and grilled chicken voluntarily. I enjoyed packing my lunch and making sure my meals were healthy.

And, for the first time ever in my life, I had women interested in me. I also made more friends and cared about my appearance.

However, once I hit college, I backslid on my diet and fitness. With the anxiety of a new place, I let the stress drive me to eating. For me, the freshman 15 was the freshman 30. I ballooned to 185 pounds, which was huge on my 5'6" frame.

I know that my weight affected my social life as well. I struggled to get dates when I was at my highest weight. It affected my ability to be a healthy and happy college student in the "prime of my life."

Again, I reached a mental limit. One night I weighed myself at a friend's house when I went to use the bathroom. I was shocked I had let myself get that big.

I was tired of being tired (literally, since I was out of shape). I got my butt in gear. I played racquetball with a friend, began to bike, walked, and cut back on my eating significantly.

When I went to graduate school, I was down forty pounds and felt great. It had given me a new outlook on life and I experienced all the benefits of health and fitness.

Now, I'm 37. And, although my weight has fluctuated here and there, I've never gotten close to 185 again. I've settled into a routine of moderately low carb eating and a fitness schedule that involves running and intense interval training.

The struggle, however, remains real. I still count calories every day and have been since 2008. I know that if I stop, I'll get back into old patterns. I avoid sugary drinks and always check calories when I go to a restaurant. My friends think I'm obsessed, but it's just to keep my fit and healthy lifestyle.

I tell people this: I've been fat and I've been thin. Thin is much better. When I'm thinner, I feel better about myself, I get more attention and respect from others, and I'm able to live life to the fullest physically.

If you are obese, you are missing out. I promise you. While you have to love yourself as you are, you also need to love yourself to make yourself your best. This book will help you reach your best physical self.

- Jonathan

CHAPTER 1

ENJOY YOUR FOOD AND ENJOY YOUR LIFE

This was actually one of the last tips I wrote, but I put it at chapter one because I wanted to emphasize its importance. Fundamentally, if you want to lose weight, you need to understand and live this secret principle. What is it?

Enjoy food. Yes. Enjoy food. That is the big "secret." I am healthy, in great shape, and happy. I have learned a thing or two about weight loss, exercise, and eating, since I began writing my tips in 2009. This tip is so important, that instead of putting at the end, I decided to start the book with it. To enjoy food is so fundamental that it has shaped the way I view both life and food.

When I first wrote this chapter, I analyzed my relationship with food. Why is it so rocky? Ever since I was 11 or 12, as I mentioned in the introduction, I remember being driven by food. Eastern philosophy uses the word "tethered" to describe my relationship with food. Whether I have been overeating or dieting, the result has been that my mind has been focused on food, food, and more food.

As I previously mentioned, in 5th grade I took a field trip all over the local area, visiting steamboats and other historical sites. I even got to drive a steamboat. However, I barely remember caring about any of that. All that concerned me was the eating. My brother and I went over the itinerary in our minds before, during, and after the trip, and the focus was entirely on the places where we ate.

I still remember them: Western Sizzlin Steak House, and the John Henry Restaurant (both closed). This was the same period the school cooks knew me on a first name basis, because I was such an enthusiastic customer. In 8th grade the process continued. I took a school trip to Florida, and all mattered to me was that I had 30 (yes, 30) packets of Sprees stocked up for the trip to and from.

I certainly wasn't packing light for that trip! I can name other examples too. I have been a yo-yo dieter since I discovered the concept of a diet as a freshman in high school. My weight fluctuated wildly in high school, from a fairly lean 170 to an overweight 185. At every peak and valley, I often felt anxiety and guilt about eating.

You would think that all this obsession with food would mean I actually appreciate food. Those who overeat know this isn't true. In fact, the opposite is true. Most of the time when I eat, I go into an altered state, a food trance. I do not savor anything. I scarf down food as quickly as possible, with as little enjoyment as necessary.

As I eat, I physically feel my body tensing up. When I finish, the tension is relieved somewhat, and I feel bloated and my mind becomes foggy. This is not enjoying food. So, what is the answer? After reading various books, I think the answer to this is mindfulness.

I have been reading about mindfulness lately, after I picked up Jon Kabat-Zinn's *Wherever You Go, There You Are.*

Mindfulness is simply being present and aware, and non-judgmental, in the moment. It is living in the present to the fullest extent possible. This got me thinking about mindfulness and eating. Why do I go into a narrow-focused trance state every time I eat?

Why do I look forward to meals, yet scarf them down so quickly as not to really enjoy them? Most of us have trouble enjoying the present moment in all areas of life, but food is one area that I really struggle to simply "be present" in the moment.

I decided to buy *Mindful Eating* by Jan Chozen-Bays. I highly recommend it. It has made me realize I probably haven't really enjoyed a meal in a long, long, time. According to Chozen-Bays, mindful eating is being aware of the experience we have while eating. It is being attuned to our hunger and experience of food.

Mindful eating has us asking questions such "why am I hungry?" and "how am I hungry?" It has me paying attention to the tastes, textures, flavors, colors, smells, and experience of a meal.

Mindful eating has taught me to slow down and actually enjoy a meal, and to live in the experience of eating a great piece of food or glass of liquid. Yes, we can even savor water! According to Bays, mindfulness is "the best seasoning!"

Being mindful is extremely simple, but difficult to sustain. Our minds are bombarded by random thoughts and worries. When we try to focus on the present, our mind brings us to our past ("you ate too much of that last time!") or the future ("you might get fat if you eat this").

Fortunately, Chozen-Bays provides some tips to eat more mindfully. I am listing a few below, but I highly recommend you read her book, or at the very least a book about general mindfulness.

1. Focus on Your Breathing - This is a way to be generally mindful. Pause wherever you are right now and sit, stand, or lie down comfortably. Next, focus on your breath. Just be aware of the sensation of breathing, the feeling, sound, etc.

Continue doing this. When you get a random thought, acknowledge it, and move back to focusing on breathing. After doing this for a few moments, you will find yourself being more aware.

You will see, hear, feel, taste, and smell things you didn't before. Your field of vision will get wider. Colors will become more vibrant. The entire experience will become more vivid and meaningful. You will go from semi-zombie to fully conscious.

2. Eat Slowly - It might sound obvious, but slowing down is key. This can be accomplished a variety of ways, including by chewing more slowly and placing the eating utensil down between bites.

In order to fully appreciate the intricate flavors, smells, and textures of a meal, slowing down is absolutely crucial. If you find yourself mindlessly eating, slow down a little more. Use the breathing technique to refocus on the present moment.

3. Be Non-Judgmental - This seems counter-intuitive to most dieters. They believe that they have to judge food and the entire eating experience. After all, it is food that has gotten them in the mess!

Actually, the opposite is true. Most dieters are so anxious about the past and future that they have never actually enjoyed a meal.

So, instead of feeling full and satisfied after eating a delicious meal, the dieter is too busy worrying about what the scale will say tomorrow.

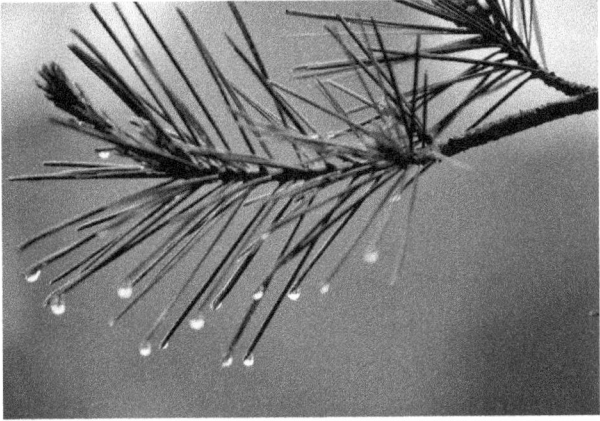

The first time I tried some of these techniques was amazing. I realized my problem has not been enjoying food too much, but not enjoying it enough! Chozen-Bays mentions that it is okay to play with your food, so instead of eating at the table or in front of the TV, my wife and I decided to "have a picnic" in front of the fireplace.

We put a blanket down and faced each other. The cat sat in between us, while the flames warmed us. My wife made spare ribs with a tomato sauce, over whole wheat noodles. We enjoyed our meal slowly, and became aware of the experience. We talked a little, but left plenty of time for just being aware.

It is difficult to be mindful if you are talking a lot. Mindfulness is being aware, not necessarily thinking. The flavors and experience came alive! Each bite was a little different, and the blend of spices and texture made it a great experience. While doing this, I became attuned to my stomach, and realized that I was full fairly quickly. I even left some food for later.

As I looked up out the window during the meal, I noticed a strong orange and blue hue shining in, as the sun was setting outside our house. I realized that this is the way a meal was meant to be.

Not only did the food come alive, but the entire experience did. The alternative, staring at a TV screen while inhaling the meal, now strikes me as a total waste of time.

As you read this, you might be wondering how this will affect weight gain and loss. The point of mindful eating is not about losing or gaining weight, in the sense that it is about enjoying both food and the moment. However, so far it has had a very positive impact on my weight.

One principle of eating mindfully is to recognize different types of hunger, and satisfy them. Eating fully aware is a great way to satisfy the types of hunger that we have. My results have been very encouraging.

The experience of eating mindfully satisfies my needs. I recognize when I am full more quickly. Enjoying the food actually renders it more satisfying, so I don't have to stuff myself just to feel as if I am "getting something" from it.

Who would have guessed the dieter and overeater suffer from the same problem? Neither enjoys food enough.

Both are "tethered" to food, and neither appreciates the moment of eating. For most of us, perhaps the greater issue is not being mindless about food, but being mindless about all of life.

Being mindlessly obsessed with food, whether by overeating or undereating, is not the answer, but rather, being present in the eating moment, and fully enjoying our food, is what has put eating in perspective for me.

Today enjoy your next meal mindfully.

- David

CHAPTER 2

GET EXCITED (AND SIX WAYS TO DO IT)

As I begin to consider the lifestyle changes and actions that have helped me lose weight, I think I should really start from the beginning, which is GET EXCITED.

I admit that I my weight has fluctuated over the years, and one very important factor that has allowed me to lose excess weight (and keep it off) is to get excited about losing weight and getting in shape.

Experts tell us that our mind doesn't necessarily know the difference between what we think is true, and what is true.

If we get excited about weight loss, then we are constantly telling ourselves how we will lose weight and reach our goal! When this excitement fades, it becomes more difficult to lose weight, because our mind is no longer able to think as positively as when we started.

I am not saying that every moment has to leave you exclaiming "boy, eating broccoli instead of ice cream is awesome...I sure prefer sulfur-containing chemicals to sugar," because that is not realistic. But, if weight loss and getting in shape is tantamount to painful torture for you, then I am guessing that losing weight is not going to be easy.

I believe that when beginning to lose weight, it is important to start out excited and fired-up. In a later chapter, I speak about developing healthy eating and fitness habits, since excitement fades, but starting out, I find that I need to be excited, to get over the initial struggles and challenges of losing weight.

In high school and college, I found that the social benefits of weight loss motivated me the most (i.e. my dating life was a basic behavioral experiment: it was better when I was thin...sometimes non-existent when I was fat!). As odd as it sounds, I am almost nostalgic for those summer days when I was thirty pounds overweight, struggling to even run 10, 100 yard sprints, drenched with sweat and embarrassingly out-of-breath.

It is not that I am some sort of masochist and yearn for the pain, but rather I remember how hopeful and excited I was to start anew during those moments. Because of the excitement, those memories are etched positively into my mind.

I hope that if you are reading this, you are at least mildly excited about weight loss. However, here are some of my ideas for getting excited about weight loss.

1. Focus on your reason behind getting healthy (e.g. looking better, improving your social life, being alive for the grandchildren, etc.), and don't let yourself forget these reasons.

Keep your goal in your mind and if you have to, continually remind yourself of the reason for your excitement (see below).

2. To keep yourself excited, remind yourself of the reasons for weight loss. One tool I use is Google Calendar. Every morning, this calendar program sends me a reminder of my daily agenda. I include

weight loss reminders (including reasons I want to lose weight) on my daily reminders.

3. Work with others to generate excitement. Talk it up with friends, family members, and even co-workers. Go shopping for healthy food together. Meet for coffee and discuss your progress. Exercise together.

I find that I do much better when I have someone to work with (this will be expanded in another tip), and part of this is because both (or all) of us help keep the other(s) excited.

4. Start a weight loss or fitness blog. Is there a more perfect, modern, way to "talk" with thousands of people about your weight loss efforts, in order to stay excited? Even if very few people are reading your story, at least you are writing it!

However, one thing about weight loss blogs is that you have to make time for it if you want to succeed. There is a veritable "boneyard" of abandoned weight-loss blogs out there that attest to the reality that weight loss blogs aren't always maintained. And make sure you actually focus more on losing weight than writing.

5. Try morning affirmations. Every morning, say out loud, the kind of day you want to have. State it positively, make it realistic, and remind yourself of your goal.

For example, you might say "Today I will eat less than 2000 calories, and exercise for at least 30 minutes, because I want to look good for Mary's wedding." By saying this, you are training your brain to believe it!

6. Try night affirmations. Every night before bed, list out loud a few things you are grateful for that happened during the day related to your weight loss.

Personally, I recommend expressing how grateful you are for people and things in every area in your life, but this article is focused on weight loss.

It is as simple as listing a few things that you did well, or that pleased you (if you can't think of any, keep trying!). For example, you might say, "I ate well, felt thinner, and had a chance to meet with my friends and talk about our weight loss strategies."

Don't dwell on the day's negatives, even if there were negatives, but be grateful for the positives.

This is not to say you should ignore where you have stumbled, because you need to be aware of mistakes to correct them in the future, but I am sure that you are already aware of the day's errors, so this exercise is meant to focus on the good things.

Today get excited about your weight loss journey! You are becoming a healthier version of yourself!

- David

CHAPTER 3

GET MOVING (ALL THE TIME)

I will speak about exercise later, but what I am about to say is pretty important too: if possible, move every chance you get, i.e. keep moving at all times and all places.

Studies show that thin people fidget more than overweight people, even moving up to two hours more in a day than non-fidgeters (3).

This means that thin fidgeters are moving a lot more in a day than their fatter, less fidgety, friends. Perhaps there is a silver lining to being hyper. At any rate, there are many ways to squeeze extra movement (and therefore calorie burning) into your average day, some which are listed below (but you should come up with some creative ways of your own):

- Take the stairs instead of the elevator.

- Instead of circling around looking for a parking spot at a store, park as far out as possible, and walk.

- When you go shopping, keep moving in the store, and move quickly; also avoid leaning on the cart for support.

- Walk to stores, places, etc., that are within walking distance.

- Get out and do activities with family and friends; In other words, choose family activities that actually require activity (for example, you could go to a pumpkin patch to pick pumpkins, instead of staying inside and watching a show on Netflix you've already seen ten times).

- Stand and move at work (you may have to get creative, depending on your line of work). As a teacher, I try to move a lot when I teach; it keeps the kids interested and allows me to burn more calories. During planning periods I try to take multiple trips to run errands instead of one.

- When waiting for someone or something, don't sit; get out and walk

- Pace while you talk on the phone or do another activity.

- Get creative!! Come up with your own ideas and put them to use.

Remember, movement is exercise. Be as active as you possibly can. I will talk more about pedometers, but most experts recommend taking 10,000 steps a day if you are trying to get fit and lose weight. I try to shoot for 10,000 or more steps daily in addition to whatever steps I get during formal exercise.

I take this pretty seriously, and even pace around my classroom during planning periods if I need more steps, cleaning desks and such. I took the most steps when I was in Washington D.C. on a student trip.

Also, one day when I subbed in a kindergarten classroom, and ran later that afternoon I nearly set a record. I took over 22,000 steps on each of these days, the equivalent of about a 10-12 mile walk!

Today start moving more! Any bit of extra movement counts.

- David

Chapter 4

Work With Friends

It is important to work with friends if you want to lose weight. Let me explain this using a story.

A few years ago, I taught for a public school that had a very successful football program (usually ranked number one in the state in their division). Despite being a rural school, they consistently dominated in football.

When I read some of their literature over the summer, I looked at some of the things they recommended for the student athletes. One of the suggestions was "talk football," that is, basically they were expected to help each other out: when hanging out with friends, the coaches wanted the athletes to think about and bring up the topic of football.

I think this is a little extreme, since students have a lot of other things to worry about besides football, including academics, but I understand the point, which is that if you want to be successful at something, and stick with it, it helps to work together, share ideas, and generate excitement together.

This illustrates an important point about losing weight and keeping it off, that you must work with friends.

I have found that weight loss is easier if I have friends and family helping me out, working with me to lose weight and be healthy. This includes sharing ideas, providing support, generating excitement, and giving mutual aid to stay on the path.

If you think about it, it makes a lot of sense: if you value something, it is likely your family and friends value it as well, which is likely one reason why your friends and family are your friends and family.

This is why I suggest asking your family and friends for at least a basic level of support (no sabotaging) and even investigating to see if your friends and family might make good formal or informal weight loss "partners." It is important to have support, and people that you can "talk weight loss" and "talk health" with.

My brother and I do this all the time. We talk about a lot of things on a daily basis, since we have a lot in common, whether on the phone, online, or in person.

We frequently discuss health and weight loss. This includes discussing the latest studies, news, recipes, insights, and so forth. It really helps both of us to stay on the path by simply "talking shop" on a regular basis, because it keeps the ideas and motivations fresh.

If you don't have anybody to do this with offline, there are plenty of us who will "talk shop" with you, and support you, online.

Also, if there are people in your life actively sabotaging your efforts, you should give them a chance to get on board (nicely), but if they continue sabotaging you, it may be time to find new friends, or at least hang out less with the people who bring you down.

Human nature is such that "misery loves company." If you get your life together, your friends whose lives are out of control may resent your success.

Ideally, you can nicely get them on board through inspiration and encouragement. However, some people simply can't see past their jealousy.

Basically, it is important to find individuals to help you lose weight. These may be family, friends, or even online friends you meet on a weight loss forum. Either way, supportive and like-minded friends will make your task easier.

Today connect with some friends about your weight loss. Offer your support and ask them for theirs!

- David

CHAPTER 5

KNOW HOW TO "GO OFF" PROPERLY

Life happens, so you need to know how to "go off" your diet properly. Sometimes, it is very difficult to stick to a weight loss plan, because it seems like almost every day "something special" happens that just begs us to get off track. It could be a co-worker's birthday cake at work, a holiday like Christmas, your husband bringing home some doughnuts someone gave him at work and so forth.

It seems like there is some sort of homemade treat in the teacher's lounge almost every day of the week! There is nothing wrong with allowing yourself to "go off" occasionally, since sustaining and losing weight should be a long term lifestyle change, not a fad diet. However, because we are talking about a long term plan, going off every other day is not a good idea. I think it is important to have a perspective about "going off." First, it is important to ask yourself two questions:

1. <u>Should I go off?</u> - Like I just mentioned, you can find a reason to abandon your health plan just about every day. You can probably think of hundreds of reasons to abandon your diet right now. So, when contemplating "going off" for a day or any period, you first have to decide if it is worth it. I tend to allow myself to go off when it truly is a "one shot" type of thing, like a birthday cake for a fellow employee or major holiday, like Christmas or Easter. These are occasional, and will not lead to a chain reaction. However, I do not allow myself to go off for lengthy periods (like extended vacations), minor holidays, or for regular activities (like when I work at a school sports events, which when I originally wrote this chapter was a two to three times a week occurrence). So, first you need to decide if it really is worth going off your diet/health plan. And next...

2. <u>If I do go off, how am I going to deal with it?</u> - If you decide to "go off" you need to decide how you are going to do it. There is a big difference between

consuming 3000 calories and consuming 6000 calories on your "off day." The former may be a break-even day for you if you were active, while the latter could easily result in you gaining a pound of fat, if the day was a particularly inactive one. Basically, being on a health plan means controlling yourself to some degree on your off days. Here are a few ways I control my chosen splurge days:

A. *Don't go completely off* - I try to never go completely nuts when I go off. For example, I haven't drunk a regular soft drink or any other full-calorie pop or sugary drink in probably fifteen years. I know that if I drink a lot of Coke with my dinner, I could easily add 500+ pointless calories to my day, whether it is an off-day or not. If I feel like a dessert, I will try to get a "no sugar added" dessert, or share a dessert dish with others, or, if the urge for a dessert is not strong, just get a coffee instead. Last night, I went off, at the Golden Corral Buffet, because I was finishing up my vacation/visit with family. I consumed 3000 calories for the day, but I still lost weight mathematically speaking, and part of the reason is that I kept my "going off" day under control. Fitday, My Fitness Pal, or other calorie tracking software will help with this.

B. *Exercise more on splurge days* - Since weight loss and gain is ultimately a math formula (see Appendix B), if you know you are going to consume more calories on a splurge day, then it makes sense to burn more calories that day. For this reason, I try to get more activity on the days I decide to splurge. This means exercising a little longer at the Y, weight-lifting harder, running that extra mile outside, or even taking a long walk after eating. Yesterday, I applied these principles. I lifted at the Y and ran outside before eating my large meal, and then walked after eating. All-in-all, I burned 3600 calories, ahead 600 for the day. I still left full and certainly felt like I splurged, but blunted the damage.

Today, get a plan together for when you "go off" and stick to it!

- David

Chapter 6

Know Your Menus

You must know your menus, because I don't believe that fad or temporary diets are beneficial. It is essential to develop an overall health plan that includes eating right, exercising, and living moderately (and if you are overweight, losing weight). I think we have to avoid getting stuck in a "diet bubble" when you can successfully lose weight in a narrow or controlled environment, but can't make it work outside of this.

Basically, I am saying that fad diets and severe restrictions are successful for a short while, but not over the long haul. This is perhaps another chapter in itself, but I'm trying to make the point that if you are trying to be healthy in the long term you need to be able to eat healthily when you eat out, and merely avoiding eating out doesn't seem to me to be a very practical option.

Let's face it, you will have to eat out at some point in your life. Avoiding it may work in the short term, but in the long term it is essential to have a plan for eating out. Know your menus!

First, let me say I don't eat out too frequently for dietary and budgetary reasons, but I eat out a few times a week with friends and family.

My personal experience here is just one example of why it is good to have a plan when eating out, even if you don't do it too frequently, because for most Americans, chances to eat out are plentiful.

My best advice from experience is to **check out a restaurant's nutritional information before going out** or on your phone while you are there. Research the menu choices so that you are able make a fully-informed choice.

Walk in all restaurants armed with the knowledge of what you should, and shouldn't, eat, from their menu. Most restaurants post nutritional information online, making the task relatively easy. If a restaurant doesn't post information, then use your head or check out websites and apps that estimate information.

Generally pick items that you would eat at home if you are on a health program, and avoid the foods you would avoid on that same program. However, sometimes the task is tricky, because restaurants have a way of adding hidden fat and calories.

Below is a brief rundown of what to get and avoid when you eat out. It is just a sampling, but it illustrates what I mentioned above: I have done my research.

Also, I should note that it is easier to avoid being trapped into eating at a bad restaurant when you pick up food and bring it home, because you can stop at multiple places if need be.

Also, I should mention, that if you are eating out, you may have trouble actually remembering what you ate when you get home and decide to evaluate how the meal impacted your diet.

As I suggest in a later chapter, if you think you will have trouble remembering what you ate, take a picture with your phone of your plate. This is especially helpful if you are tracking your calories after eating at a buffet.

If you are eating at a bad restaurant because your friends or family have insisted on it, and there are no negotiations...just do your best and maybe consider it an "off day" if it is really bad!

My basic "eating out rules" include avoiding sandwiches if possible, since buns and breads often add a lot of calories and carbs. I avoid pasta dishes for the same reasons.

I never drink full calorie drinks, and I try to avoid desserts entirely. I do allow myself lower carb options like steak, chicken wings, shrimp, etc.

Getting lower calorie vegetables as sides (broccoli, green beans, asparagus) versus higher calorie sides (mashed potatoes, macaroni and cheese, French fries) will save you a lot of calories. I also try to avoid the rolls and other bread products that come with meals.

Hamburger, Fish, and Chicken Fast Food Places – I generally recommend avoiding these places. At many places, a sandwich, drink, fries and drink can cost you a lot of calories. As of this publication, a Big Mac (530), Large Fries (510), and Large Coke (280) will set you back 1320 calories. You add a refill of Coke and you are out 1600 calories. If you are a woman trying to lose weight that might be the maximum number of calories you should consume in a day. One option is to ask for lettuce instead of a bun, and use that as a wrap. That will save you about 150 calories depending on the sandwich. Getting diet soda or water will save you more. I usually just get a ten piece chicken nugget meal, which fills me up for less than the calories of a sandwich.

Chinese Buffets - If you love Chinese buffets like I do, you have to be careful when choosing foods. I suggest going for dishes that aren't deep fried. I tend to get the shrimp, garlic green beans, crab, and other lower carb/lower calorie dishes. Be sure to watch your portions. It is very easy to underestimate what you are eating.

Pizza Places - These places are challenging. I would say avoid eating pizza on a regular basis. The best option would be a thin crust, a whole wheat option, or if a place offers it, something lower carb. Also, cheese is a better option than one that is loaded with a lot of meats. Pizza is by its nature caloric and high carb, so be careful.

Coffee Shops - Avoid the "fancy" drinks, which usually add a lot of hidden calories. A Starbucks Pumpkin Spice Latte can set you back 510 calories! To give you some perspective, I can eat a ten piece Chicken McNugget at McDonalds with two sauce packets for those calories. At coffee places, I usually get a good, bold, caffeinated coffee, and add some cream and Stevia, which I bring myself. Most places also have sugar-free syrups.

Fried Chicken Places - I avoid these places. It is impossible to make a "light" piece of fried chicken. For example a three piece meal at KFC with mashed potatoes, macaroni and cheese, biscuit, and Coke will put you back 1460 calories. I suggest getting chicken tenders and sticking to vegetable sides (like green beans).

Wings and Pub Food Places – Chicken wings with a non-sugary sauce can be a good high protein and low carb option. Getting an eight piece chicken wing dish with a hotter, non-sugar sauce, will cost you about 650 calories. Eight wings, eaten slowly enough, should easily fill you up, and this doesn't require a side dish.

Sub Sandwich Places - Many sub places advertise how great their bread is. And their breads do taste great. However, they often add a lot of calories and carbs to any meal a sub place. The best option is to get the subs wrapped in lettuce or in "salad form." That will save you a lot of calories and carbs.

Mexican – It is easy for calories to add up in these places because tortilla chips are very caloric, and many places give them away for free before your meal. For example, that little bag of chips that comes with that tiny container of cheese at Taco Bell? It will set you back 310 calories. The basket of chips at your local Mexican restaurant has about 600 calories. I suggest limiting your intake of tortilla chips and tortillas, limiting rice, and focusing on non-fried foods. Fajitas are a good option, if you focus on the meat and vegetables and limit your tortilla intake.

Higher Quality Fast Food – Places like Chipotle offer higher quality foods, but that doesn't necessarily mean the food is lighter. For example, a Barbacoa burrito with rice, pinto beans, sour cream, cheese, and salsa, with a side of chips and salsa will cost you 1635 calories, or what you may be shooting for in an entire day. I personally get a "bowl" which automatically cuts out the tortilla (300 calories and 40+ carbs), and I ask for half brown rice, cutting my calories by 105. I avoid cheese and sour cream, although I do like guacamole.

Today commit to looking up nutritional information online before you eat out, and making choices accordingly.

- David

CHAPTER 7

VARY YOUR EXERCISE ROUTINE

Before I talk about how to vary your exercise routine, I think we all agree that getting a lot of exercise (within reason) is important, so I am assuming that if you are interested in losing weight, you are already exercising.

If you are not, then start...right now! I have purposely skipped over adding "exercise" as a tip since I assume it is obvious. Maybe I am wrong.

Why is exercising obvious? Well, I just can't imagine hunter and gatherer man, or even ancient civilized man (having discovered agriculture) sitting around all day doing nothing. Humans are meant to move, not sit around in front of a rectangle-shaped box all day (whether a TV or computer monitor), or waste away in a cubicle.

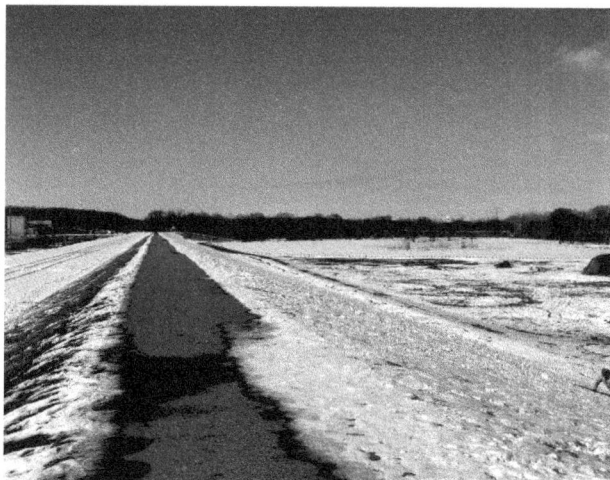

The "problem" is that in our modern Western world, we don't have to exercise for survival, so it is easy to avoid exercise, and get bored with it quickly.

I know what it is like to get sick of exercising and just give up, because I have done it before. However, I think there are ways to avoid the boredom.

I have found that when it comes to sticking with an exercise program, varying my routine is very helpful, even essential.

I cannot go to the YMCA every other morning at 5:00 AM and hop on an elliptical machine for forty minutes, repeating this endlessly for months.

If you can, then I offer my sincere congratulations, because I wish I could do that. For me to stay interested, I have to shake things up now and then. Below is what I typically do to vary my intense workouts.

Note that I try to lift weights three times a week, which means I usually set foot at the YMCA three days a week, but that doesn't always mean I work out there aerobically that many times.

- I run inside at the YMCA, usually with music playing. Studies show that listening to music allows you to work out longer.

- I change songs on my MP3 player regularly, so as to avoid boredom.

- If at the YMCA, some days I run eight miles, and do twenty minutes on the elliptical machine, or some sort of combo of running and elliptical machine. I typically shoot for the calorie equivalent of eight miles. If the weather is warmer, I run around the housing development outside the Y.

- I admit that by March I am very sick of the Y, and will do anything to run outside (I have even run on snow before). So, when the weather is remotely nice, I run outside at a state park, bike path, flood wall, school track, cemetery, or wherever I can. Exercising outside is a great way to vary your routine!

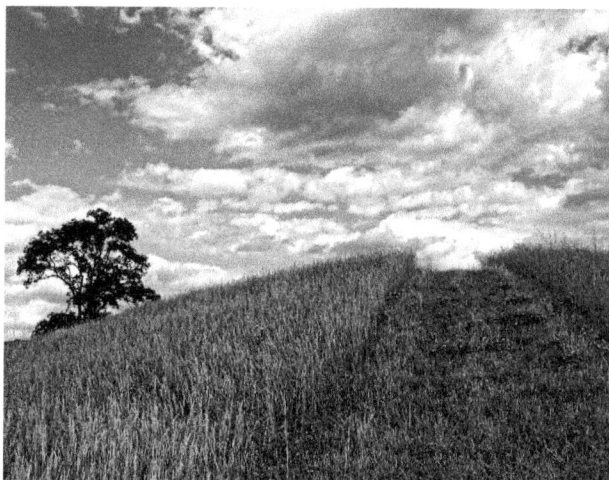

- When I run at the school track where I grew up, I run "outside" the track, over the hills, basically taking the cross-country route.

This keeps it interesting, instead of circling a black oval for an hour. My old football coach called this a "country mile."

- When I run outside, I try to take in the sights, smells, and sounds of nature, which makes the time pass more quickly (this is called "mindfulness," being completely present in the moment).

I can tell you all about the changes in nature and temperature, because I am enjoying being outside. Also, studies show that exercising in fresh air is effective in combating mild depression!

- Some days I like to run alone, to gather my thoughts. Other days, chatting with a friend or family member is my preference.

- Occasionally I will use the rowing machine, or a stationary bike when at the YMCA, but often only briefly in combination with running or elliptical.

- When I run after my job I follow the bike path in varying directions. If I want some variety, I will explore new side streets, head to the local park, or even take off on a back road.

- I also go hiking and walking regularly, which creates a change of scenery, but the above ideas refer to intense aerobic activity, which I find the most difficult to stay interested in.

As you can tell, I like running, but honestly, I hate treadmills. The surest way for me to get bored very quickly is to run on a treadmill. We are all different I suppose.

Before I close this chapter, I want to mention that exercise alone isn't going to help you lose much weight. Most people just eat more to compensate. So, while exercise is essential to any health improvement program, it must be paired with calorie restriction if you want to lose weight.

Today think of new exercises you can try to stay interested in your exercise routine.

- David

CHAPTER 8

MUSCLES MAKE YOU A CALORIE BURNING MACHINE

To weight-lift and build muscle should be a part of any serious weight loss or health program.

Why? Not only does building muscle make you look trim and fit, but it increases your metabolism every minute of the day. This is because the bigger your muscles are, the more energy it takes to feed them, even when you are not using them.

One study showed that every pound of muscle you gain increases your basal metabolic rate by 37.5 calories (4). Since in that same study participants gained an average of three pounds of muscle in six weeks, this means by the study's end, they burned

112.5 calories more per day than when they began, just by simply existing.

All things equal, this extra metabolic boost theoretically would result in almost twelve pounds of extra fat lost in a year. So you can see it is important to build muscle!

I have lifted weights since I was in high school. Back then, I lifted in a dungeon of a weight room with old, torn-up, carpeting and rusty free weights, with heavy metal music frequently blaring. However, occasionally they would put oldies on, and I recall hearing Elvis Presley's "In the Ghetto" for the first time down there.

I remember coaches giving shaky advice, insisting that we only do incline bench press, because "you aren't lying on your back when you block someone in football." Last I checked, we weren't lying at an incline when we blocked someone either, something one of the younger coaches often pointed out. Oh well. I also remember guys who would work their biceps and nothing else. I regularly skipped squats because I hated them, and I even skipped whole days of lifting because hanging out with girls struck me as more fun.

One time I was riding in the back of a friend's pick-up truck with my brother and some girls, and our football coach saw us, even though we were supposed to have just finished up lifting. Ahh memories!

The point is that building muscle has nothing to do with the awkward memories of hanging around meatheads all day. There are many ways to build muscle that don't even involve picking up a dumbbell. Push-ups, chin-ups, squats, crunches, triceps dips, and other exercises make gaining muscle easy, even if you can't afford a gym membership.

There are many websites that have free information about exercises you can do with or without free weights or weight machines. It is beyond the scope of this book to provide you with detailed descriptions of exercises, but there is a lot of free information out there.

I mainly do resistance exercises that involve my body and some basic dumbbell work (and unlike in my adolescence, I don't skip sessions to hang out with girls). I try to do some type of muscle building exercise three times a week, every other day if possible.

I suggest programs like Beachbody's Insanity, P90x, and Asylum if you want some good programs that combine muscle building with aerobic exercise that don't involve a lot of time in the gym.

There are a lot of myths about muscle building. You don't have to "bulk up" like bodybuilders to gain muscle. Women and men both can gain muscle without much change in appearance.

To get a "ripped" or "bulked" look requires a lot of training, and in some cases, illegal substances. I prefer the lean and toned look that I get from using Insanity and other programs.

The bottom line is that if you aren't building muscle, you are failing to use a powerful tool that will help your body burn extra calories.

Today explore ways you can build muscle that are in line with your weight loss and fitness goals.

- David

CHAPTER 9

KNOWLEDGE IS POWER

If you are really interested in something, what do you do? You probably get educated and get informed about it, and maybe even obsess a little. Think of something you are interested in. Maybe it is music, sports, a TV show, religion, or even your prize insect collection (it takes all types, right?).

Now, think of all the information you probably have about this subject, the books, magazines, web pages, and so forth. Why have you acquired all of this information? Because you care about the subjects, and you want to know as much as possible. Get educated!

If you care about weight loss and health, then it makes sense to educate yourself about these too. I am not saying you have to buy hundreds of weight loss books to equal your comic book collection, or buy as many health magazines as you have Rolling Stone mags, but if you want to be successful at losing weight, you have to be knowledgeable, and probably more importantly, develop a thirst for knowledge about health and wellness.

I started reading about health back in 1992, when I was 14. Jonathan checked out *Dr. Lendon Smith's Diet Plan for Teenagers* from the library, and from there I bought other books related to fitness, health, and alternative medicine. I looked forward to book shopping with my parents. I remember reading health books right before bedtime (after a busy day of school and football).

Unfortunately, I didn't always follow the good advice contained in these books (some books contained a mix of good and bad advice), **but at least I had the knowledge to fall back on, knowledge which I continued to have in the back-of-my-head, even when I was making bad choices**.

I believe that by educating ourselves, and staying informed, we place ourselves ahead of the curve.

Weight loss and good health are difficult to maintain in a society with so many unhealthy temptations, so any advantage is helpful. Knowledge always provides an advantage. A good example is when I read recently in *Prevention* that diets high in monounsaturated fats are associated with greater weight loss, specifically belly fat loss.

I now eat more peanuts, and other nuts, and use olive oil more often. I always knew that these fats were healthy, but I now know that they are helpful in shedding harmful belly fat.

In high school, I made a hand-drawn, make-shift chart that listed all the healthy things I wanted to accomplish. It contained a table of things like "don't eat after 6:30 PM," and "stretch at least 3 minutes" and I weighted each one so that all of them added up to 100%.

At the end of the day, I gave myself a grade out of one hundred. It was needlessly complicated and I didn't stick to it very long. Nonetheless, I benefited from the research and reading I did to make that chart.

I just can't stress enough the importance of being informed. I view weight loss like being in a battle. The foe, body fat, is extremely powerful. I recall reading in a health magazine in the 1990s that if a person does not lose his or her excess body fat at puberty, then he or she has only a 1 in 35 chance of getting thin. You could be that 1 person in 35, but you darn well better have powerful weapons at your disposal!

This is where knowledge comes in. If you can attack your weight loss from multiple "fronts" then you are likely to do better. If restricting calories by eating rice cakes for every meal is all you got, then you are in serious trouble. If you are making use of all the tips in this book, then you are much better armed and likely to succeed at weight loss. However, how would you know about these ideas if you aren't informing yourself?

So how do you get educated? I used to read a lot of books and magazines, and I still do, but the internet contains a wealth of good information (but some bad information too, so beware!!). Generally mainstream news sites like CNN, Fox News, Yahoo News, Google News, etc., have health and medicine sections and are worth checking out, as new studies and information become available.

I like Reddit as a place to find and discuss helpful information. The subreddits "r/loseit" and "r/supplements" are particularly helpful and sensible.

Unfortunately, when dealing with supplements and weight loss programs there are often a lot of unproven claims about them floating on the Internet.

Wading through the fads, pyramid schemes, hype, and fringe information can be challenging, but in the end, it is worth it. Information is power, and to lose weight, you'll need that power.

Today commit to learning something new each day that can benefit your health goals.

- David

CHAPTER 10

AVOID THE WHITE STUFF

I often call sugar "the white stuff," likening it to a certain hard drug that was snorted off mirrors in the eighties.

Obviously it is nowhere near cocaine in its immediate destructiveness, but evidence suggests that as high fructose corn syrup (basically sugar) became more available in soft drinks and other foods, America and other Western countries have gotten fatter. Excess sugar intake has also been linked to an increase in diabetes, heart disease, and gout (5).

This is why to lose weight you must get rid of excess sugar in your diet. I have no qualms about saying clearly that excess sugar is bad, very bad. I try to avoid it as much as possible, although sugars occur naturally in a variety of foods and cannot (and should not) be avoided entirely.

What I am primarily speaking of here is unnaturally high-sugar, processed foods and drinks. I do allow myself sugary treats now and then, but I try to avoid a steady, high, everyday consumption of sugar and high sugar products (and this includes certain fruit juices). Get rid of the sugar!

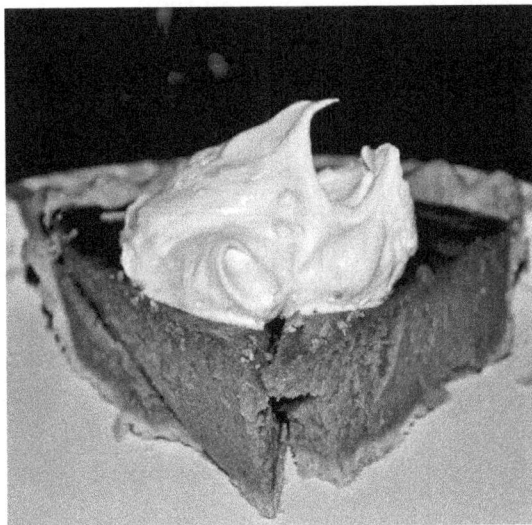

Processed sugar is a modern marvel really. I just can't imagine ancient man eating as much sugar as we do, since he didn't have the tools to extract large amounts of sugars from fruits and other sources (had you given ancient man a bushel of corn, I doubt he would have thought "hey, maybe there's high fructose syrup in there!"). Fruits and their juices truly would have been rare desserts for ancient men and women.

At least these ancient treats were sugar surrounded by nutrients and fiber, which slowed their absorption, thus preventing a blood sugar spike. Most sugary drinks consumed today are basically empty calories, or what I tend to call "pointless calories" (more on this in a second).

Have you ever looked at the ingredients in a bottle of cola? It is pretty much sugar (in the form of high fructose corn syrup), caramel coloring, some natural flavors, caffeine, and of course, carbonated water, and yet Coke and Pepsi have no problem charging you $1.50 for two liters of this stuff. It doesn't really fill you up, and if you drink it with a meal, you probably barely notice it's there.

But, if you manage to consume three large glasses of cola at a meal, you still will consume 600 calories. This is why I call calories from sugary drinks "pointless calories" because when you really look forward to a meal, or go to a restaurant, you probably do so for a steak, pizza, General Tso's Chicken, or whatever, and yet along with that you probably get 600 calories from your drink, which, if consumed six days in a week, will result in you gaining a pound for that week (600×6=3600 calories). You may not really notice the sugary drinks you consume, but other people will notice them as they cause you to slowly gain weight.

Not only does excess sugar increase your calorie consumption, it raises your blood sugar levels, creating insulin resistance, making losing weight more difficult. It also will increase your cravings for more sugar. Excess sugar is bad news, really bad news, like learning Justin Bieber released a new album (that's just a little harmless joke for all the Beliebers reading this). .

Below are some methods that I employ to try to avoid sugar. I hope that you find them helpful in your weight loss.

- Drink sugar-free drinks (like coffee, water, teas, etc.). It may take some time to get used to drinks without sugar, but give them a try. Your body will thank you. You will be amazed how much money and calories you will save if you drink water with a meal. Yep. Simple, clear, and refreshing water.

- Don't add sugar to naturally sweetened foods. For example, don't add sugar to grapefruit or applesauce.

- Don't insist that every meal has to end (or perhaps begin) with a dessert.

- When you must eat a processed sweet, go for a lower sugar option (like "no sugar added" products). See substitutes below.

One problem we face is that getting a sweet taste without sugar requires the use of artificial sweeteners, which have their own problems. Some studies show that artificial sweeteners cause people to gain weight, probably because artificial sweeteners don't really satisfy our cravings for sugar, but give us a taste for it, so most people just eat more calories elsewhere to compensate. Keep this in mind when consuming "diet" foods and drinks.

The safest artificial sweeteners seem to be sugar alcohols, like sorbitol and mannitol, which have fewer calories per gram than sugar, and don't raise blood sugar levels. They are absorbed less readily than sugars, which means sugar alcohols effectively provide even fewer calories to our bodies, but they are still caloric.

Because they are poorly absorbed, they can cause digestive disturbances in large amounts (chew a half of pack of gum with sugar alcohols to feel what I am talking about!), and are often present in candies and foods marked "no sugar added," including sugarless gum. Occasionally you can find these available in powder form.

Saccharin (aka Sweet-N-Low), usually comes in pink packets, and tastes bitter to me. It has an uneven safety record in animal studies. However, you would have to eat piles of it a day to produce the negative effects seen in animals (bladder cancer), so it is probably safe in moderate amounts.

I like the taste of Aspartame (aka Equal), which usually comes in blue packets, but it has a sketchy safety record, and the manner in which it was approved was downright shady. Apparently the FDA gets more complaints about Aspartame than just about any other food product. Even though Aspartame is a combination of the amino acids Aspartic Acid and Phenylalanine, when heated it breaks down into formaldehyde, so it can't be used in baking, although it could be used as an embalming agent I suppose.

Splenda, i.e. Sucralose, comes in yellow packets, and tastes good to me, but there are safety concerns with it as well, since it is made by chlorination (adding chlorine to the sucrose molecule). One side effect may be that it reduces the "good bacteria" in your gut. You can bake with it, which makes it nice for a variety of recipes. It is now available in generic form, but the brand name Splenda is pricey. I don't find sucralose based products as sweet as other options.

Stevia, now FDA approved as a sweetener under the name Truvia, is probably my favorite option. Other forms of Stevia besides Truvia are available, but are sold not as sweeteners, but "dietary supplements," which is how Stevia was legally sold prior to the recent FDA approval of Truvia. Stevia is usually sold as a concentrated powder, a highly purified, super-sweet, herbal extract.

It has few side effects (the Japanese use it as their primary artificial sweetener). One problem is that if you use too much, it tastes bitter, and if you are using a concentrated extract, a little goes a long way, so sometimes it is hard to figure out how much to use (25 mg is as sweet as about 4 grams of sugar). This stuff is super, super sweet. Even a little dusting is overpoweringly sweet. Finally, since we are dealing with an herbal extract, different Stevia products may taste different from each other, making cooking with it in recipes frustrating.

And you think our artificial sweeteners are a bit unsafe...the ancient Romans used lead acetate!

The bottom line is that sugar and high-sugar products are generally empty and pointless calories that can lead to quick weight gain. If you are addicted to the legal "white stuff" you may want to cut down your consumption. Your body will thank you!

Today commit to eliminating or reducing processed sugar from your diet.

- David

CHAPTER 11

IF YOU EAT GRAINS, MAKE THEM WHOLE

Whole grain products are made from the bran and endosperm of grains, whereas refined grain products contain only the endosperm. Bran is grainy and thick (think All-Bran cereal) so many people prefer the taste of refined grains, and refined meal products, like white flour.

However, whole grains contain more vitamins, minerals, phytonutrients, and fiber. Whole grains are also rich in inositol hexaphosphate, i.e. phytic acid, which preliminary research suggests may have an anti-cancer effect in cultures that consume a lot of food, by removing excess minerals from the body.

And more good news is that recent research has shown that whole grains help you lose weight, specifically the harmful belly fat that puts you at risk of heart disease. In one study, even though those consuming refined grains lost some weight too, the whole grain group experienced a steep decline in C-reactive protein, which is associated with increased risk of heart disease and diabetes. The unrefined grain group did not see a decline in this harmful protein, meaning despite losing weight, they weren't experiencing some of the health benefits normally associated with weight loss (5).

Believe it or not, whole grains don't have to taste bad, and I think whole grain foods have a meatier taste, which is why I prefer whole grain breads, pastas, and other products to their refined counterparts. Because whole grains are high in fiber, they make you feel more full, and have fewer absorbable calories than refined products.

A good example is whole wheat pasta, which has 90 calories an ounce. Refined pasta has 105 calories an ounce. The main difference is that the whole grain pasta has more fiber, and insoluble fiber calories don't get counted in the total.

So, eating four ounces of whole grain pasta will cost you 360 calories, while the regular stuff puts you back 420 calories. Thus, whole grain pasta contains 15% fewer calories, and has a lot more of the good stuff you need, like Magnesium. As I mention in a later chapter, the extra fiber alone could help you lose weight.

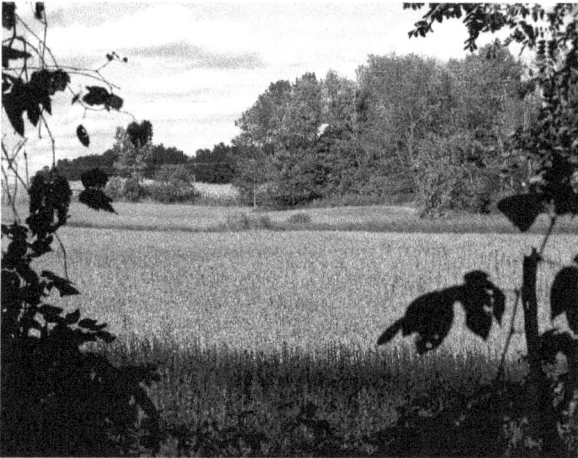

My view of whole grains is somewhat mixed overall. If you must eat grains, then going "whole" is probably the way to go. Some individuals seem to be sensitive to certain grains, like wheat and corn. Celiac disease is an example of an extreme sensitivity to wheat. I find that I feel better when I don't eat a lot of wheat or corn. Also, grains are typically high in carbohydrates, and I try to keep my carbs in the 75-

175 gram range. So, for me, I consume grains in a limited amount.

When buying whole grain products, be careful to avoid getting tricked into thinking you are getting whole grains when you aren't. Look for labels like "100% whole wheat" or "100% whole grain" or something similar. Many products will say things like "contains whole grains" (this may mean it contains one percent) or "wheat bread." Wheat bread is often just refined flour that hasn't been bleached, so it looks like whole wheat, but isn't.

The bottom line is that whole grains may take a little getting used to, but they are much healthier alternatives to refined products, and may help you lose weight by making you feel fuller, and providing fewer absorbable calories.

Today, buy some whole grain products and replace your refined grain products.

- David

CHAPTER 12

WORK HARD AND HEALTH WILL BE A HABIT

In chapter one, I mentioned it is important to get excited about weight loss, but now I am going to write a lengthy chapter about something that is at least as, if not more, important: being into health for the long haul, and turning good health into a habit.

One way to define the term habit is to consider it your "default setting," developed by years of doing something a certain way. Related to health, ask yourself this question. When you "slip" into a habit, or default way of doing things related to your health, what do you slip into? A healthy or unhealthy lifestyle? Or something perhaps in between?

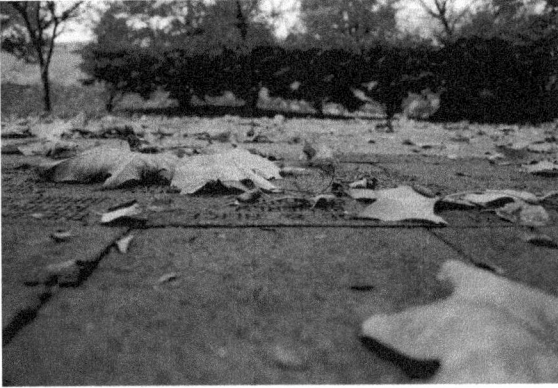

I think for most Americans, being unhealthy is certainly the default position, while being healthy is the anomaly. Wouldn't it be great if our habit, our "default setting" was healthy? Imagine the reduction in health care costs and the increase in quality of life! I hope that making health a habit is ultimately the goal of any long-term weight loss and maintenance program.

Most of us are good at temporary adjustments. We can stick to eating whole grains for a month, but a year later, will our cupboards be filled with refined grains again? Will the regular exercising last? Will you be eating those healthy recipes that excited you so much in January by the time March arrives? Will you gain back those twenty pounds and then some?

These are depressing questions, but they must be addressed, because the initial excitement about weight loss won't last forever. So how can we turn temporary good health adjustments into long-term habits?

Well...let me tell you from experience, it isn't easy. I have been "into" health since 1993, read many books, visited thousands of websites, exercised many hours, tested countless healthy recipes, and so forth, and while many healthy habits come much easier now than in 1993, it is still not always easy to "default" to healthy.

Part of the problem is that we have evolved to love sweet and fatty foods. Our bodies know that these foods contain the most calories. A creamy, sweet, food makes the older parts of our brains feel pleasure. For most of human history, the problem was not eating too much, but too little (and this is the case still in many parts of the world). Our brains still think we are living in the world of 100,000 years ago. So, with the wide availability of high calorie foods our brains crave, working hard to establish good eating and exercise habits is essential to staying healthy.

I have turned a lot of temporary health improvements into habits, so it is possible to overcome our natural desires. Very few people, myself included, are probably going to develop completely healthy habits, but I think you make yourself much more likely to lose weight, and keep it off, when you develop at least some healthy behaviors as habits. You will find that not only do you stay thinner longer, but when you do gain weight, you do so more slowly. Let me share some of my habits that I have developed (and one I just can't quite get!).

When I started drinking sugar free-drinks in 1998, it was tough. Prior to this, I assumed that sugar-free drinks weren't "manly," so I only drank ones with loads of sugar. Yeah...it makes little sense now, that somehow eating sugar and getting fat and fluffy is somehow manly, especially since having belly fat reduces testosterone levels in men. Take note guys: if you want more dates, lose weight.

At any rate, my friend Dave got into diet drinks, and when we hung out on weekends, he usually bought me what he bought, so I came to like sugar-free drinks (he got a good job right out of high school, so he usually paid!). I really haven't touched a sugared drink for years. So drinking sugar-free drinks has become a habit, i.e. my default.

I also try to avoid snack foods, like potato chips, Doritos, and tortilla chips in the house. I have kind of made this a habit. I haven't had potato chips in the house for years, nor Doritos. Regular tortilla chips (with salsa!) are a weakness of mine, and I had them in the house in the winter of 2008, and I paid for it too. I ate too many of them and gained about seven or eight pounds. But nonetheless, I tend to keep these out of the house, and this has become a habit, the default, even if I do go through some extended periods when I have them in the house.

Another example of a developed habit is eating non-fried seafood regularly. In 2004 I read that DHA, an Omega-3 fatty acid present in a lot of seafood, increases brain power. I was studying for the GRE at that time, and decided to eat a lot of white tuna and salmon, rich in DHA. Before this period, I ate some fish, mostly fried.

After learning to love seafood to prepare for the GRE, I almost always choose a seafood dish over a poultry or red meat dish. This is a habit I have kept up. I have white tuna, shrimp, and grilled salmon regularly, supplying probably three times the Omega-3 fats I got in the years previous. I am not sure if I am too much smarter, but I enjoy eating the seafood.

I have been a little more inconsistent making exercise a long-term habit, but over the last 15 years since I got into health, I have regularly exercised more often than not, but there certainly have been embarrassing periods of inactivity sandwiched between the good times. Thus, I can say exercise has become a habit, the default, even if barely.

Exercise has become more of a habit for me as I have gotten older, primarily because I like the way regular exercise makes me feel. My senior year at Ohio University I had let myself get so out-of-shape that I got winded climbing one flight of dorm stairs. That made my body (and ego) feel pretty bad, and I don't feel like going there again anytime soon. I look back now and regret that I spent over half of my college years heavy because I didn't exercise enough.

One thing I haven't been too good at is restricting calories. I would love to make a habit out of eating less. I have always had a huge appetite, even when I was younger. This is why I need an app to track my food intake. I also have to choose foods that are filling, yet not calorie dense, so I feel like I am eating quite a bit, without the calories. Eating generally healthy foods is a habit for me, but eating less of all foods is still a struggle.

How did these become habits for me? Below I detail some of the ways that I went from temporary adjustment to longer-term habit. I hope that these help you do the same.

1. <u>Care About Your Health</u> - Do you know anybody who is a talented and seasoned basketball player who hates basketball? I don't. If you don't care about your health, then you won't be able to turn temporary fixes into long-term habits. You have to make your health and well-being as big a priority as your interest in your favorite sports team or reality show. If you have time to watch a ten hour Netflix marathon, you have time to exercise.

2. <u>Focus on the Long-Term, Not Just On "Quick Fixes"</u> - Are you the guy or gal who dismisses new ideas or pretends that a brief crash diet is all you need to get back on track? Is your only concern getting in shape for bikini or football season? Then, you probably won't make long-term changes, because you aren't thinking long term. You have to care, and have to want to make a long-term lifestyle change. If a quick-fix is all you are looking for, then you won't make long-term changes.

3. <u>Keep Educating Yourself</u> - If I wasn't concerned about the effects of excess sugar on my

body, I never would have even considered lowering my intake of refined sugars. Educating ourselves about health, fitness, and weight loss is extremely important, because approaching being healthy from every possible angle makes being healthy much easier, and allows us to avoid eating and doing things that make us less healthy. For example, if you think that it is healthy to eat rice cakes and water, I can tell you that you won't (and shouldn't) develop that as a habit.

4. <u>Branch Out, Be Creative, and Try New Things</u> - How could I develop a habit of liking low-sugar foods if I wasn't even willing to try them? Convincing yourself you hate broccoli because you hated it when you were three is not a very healthy way of thinking, because preferences, and taste buds, change. I have met many people that take this view, mostly overweight people not surprisingly, who refuse to try new things, yet remaining strangely puzzled why they can never seem to lose weight. If you want to make eating more vegetables a habit, you should try every vegetable possible, find them fresh, and find tasty and healthy ways to prepare them. Don't boil broccoli, declare it awful, give up on vegetables, and reach for the nearest Twinkie.

5. <u>Sometimes Just Do What Is Right, Because It Is Right</u> - In religious and philosophical circles, we call this a virtue, fortitude. Some days you might not "feel" like avoiding the doughnuts at work, or running three miles. This is where fortitude comes in. Some days we just have to do the right thing because we know we should, and this includes being healthy. Some days you may hate the thought of working out, but you know you should, so you do. You feel better afterward, but that isn't the point: you did it because it is right, even though it is tough. Perhaps this is called toughness. Whatever you call it, this is when you really start to develop health as a habit, because you are doing what is right despite the challenges you are facing.

6. <u>Continually Keep Trying</u> - One thing I learned from high school football is that you get knocked down about every play, but you get up for the next one and carry on. My weight has fluctuated more than what is ideal over the years, but I can really see a pattern of increased success in fighting weight, and it is getting much easier. In high school, my weight usually fluctuated by 10-15 pounds in the course of a year, every year. When I lost weight in college, I remained thin for a year, then fell off, then repeated this same pattern. My senior year in college (in 2000) I

was 40 pounds overweight, but I lost it all by January of 2001. I kept it off until 2005, then I started gaining 30 pounds again slowly. I got down to a good weight by my wedding in September of 2007, and I am going strong now. My point? I am keeping the weight off longer and gaining it more slowly as I get older. Each time I slip up, I eventually get back on track, and with each new attempt to get healthy, I am further training myself, further developing my short-term healthy actions into long(er) term habits.

7. <u>Progress Incrementally</u> - One mistake dieters make is to try to make too many changes too quickly. It is easy to throw out all of your desserts and replace them with rice cakes...for about two weeks, and then, the excitement dies down, and the taste of slightly-salted cardboard...er...rice cake, becomes boring. Developing healthy habits takes time. Set small goals, and build incrementally. If you can't quite give up Twinkies, then don't. First, cut down to three a week, and go from there. There is nothing worse than stopping Twinkies cold-turkey. Making incremental changes is also important for developing an exercise routine. One mistake a friend of mine makes is to start off with guns blazing, running two miles the first day! He kills himself, is sore for a week, and tired of exercise after just one day of doing it. A more

realistic, incremental, approach would be better. As my friend Joshua Wagner told me, some days his goal is to touch the door handle at the gym! It is simple, and attainable, and he knows that once he touches that handle, he never turns back!

Weight loss and maintenance are not easy, and it will take strength, effort, and focus to get, and stay, healthy for the long haul. Keep long-term goals in focus, and over time, your temporary healthy adjustments will become longer-term habits, your "default" position.

Today do something you know is good for you even if you don't feel like it.

- David

CHAPTER 13

CUT THE CABLE AND DITCH THE NETFLIX

I may have had your interest until this point, but now you may be shaking your head. "Come on!" you may be thinking. "I'm only human, David!"

I know this is one of the most controversial things I will say about losing weight, and maybe to some people, the most extreme suggestion yet, but here goes (bearing in mind that obesity has extreme control over many people, so extreme action is sometimes needed): Cut the Cable (or, get rid of Netflix).

Yeah, I'm one of "those people," that annoying friend who brags about not having cable. It's true that

I haven't subscribed to cable since 2003, which has saved me over five thousand dollars.

One story always reminds me why not having cable not only saves me money, but may save my health. At the beginning of the 2008-2009 school year, my students were sharing their favorite television shows as an ice-breaker at the beginning of the year. One girl said, "My mom won't let us get cable because she says it will make our family fat." Her mother is probably right on. The book *Super-Sized Kids* hammers the same point home.

Watching a lot of TV is one good way to get fat. Men watch around 4:35 hours of TV a day, women, 5:14, teens, 3:21, and children 3:25. When you couple this with a nine hour work day, men are either working or watching TV 13:35 hours a day. This doesn't leave much time for physical activity, planning and cooking healthy meals, or getting a decent night's sleep (which as I point out later is essential for maintaining a healthy weight) (6).

Plus, it seems like once you plop down in front of the TV, it is very hard to get up. I know obese persons who literally work all day, get home, and sit in front of the TV all night. Then, they go to bed, sometimes also in front of a TV, repeating the process nearly seven days a week. Remember the chapter on habit? Well, spending nearly five hours doing something is a great way to make it a habit.

As time passes, this routine becomes easier and easier, because they keep gaining weight, which makes getting active that much more difficult. Some of these folks used to live very active lives, playing a lot of sports and participating in other activities, but sadly, not anymore. Hey, I know that work often wears us out, but the fastest way to get even more worn out is to sit in front of a TV for a few hours.

The negative impact of watching too much television is even greater on children. According to research presented in *Super-Sized Kids*, pre-school children who watched the most TV had the greatest increases in body fat. Another study found that the amount of television a child watches corresponds directly to the risk of developing serious health problems as an adult.

For children of normal weight, watching TV triggers a 12% drop in metabolism, whereas obese children see a 16% drop. I suspect that much of this applies to adults who watch too much TV. Additionally, we don't want our kids growing up overweight, and studies show that if we want our kids to develop healthy habits, we have to model them. We just can't tell our children that too much TV is bad, we have to show them by our actions (6).

I am not against TV, and watch it probably more than I should. However, without cable at home, I am less likely to sit in front of the TV for too long, because there often isn't much on (NBC comes in fuzzy, and ABC not at all).

A few years ago, I recall one night when I was "bored," and since there was nothing on the five channels I could get with the rabbit ears, I took a refreshing walk. Had there been something interesting on TV, it is likely I wouldn't have left the house, and wouldn't have walked those extra 4000 steps.

I also think that watching too much TV causes us to miss out on what is good and meaningful in life. I am only speaking for myself of course, but unless I am watching an exceptionally good TV program, I probably couldn't tell you much about it a week later. However, when I am active, i.e. running, hiking, golfing, walking, going to pick-your-own farms, attending festivals, visiting friends and family, sitting in the sun-room eating breakfast, going to a restaurant with family, taking tours of local attractions, and so forth, I remember these well, and can't wait until they happen again.

I feel like I have accomplished something meaningful after doing these things. I don't usually get that feeling after watching TV, although sometimes certain shows do impress me greatly. Even though most kids would probably tell you how much they love TV, and that giving up cable would be tantamount to giving up oxygen, they would probably prefer deep-down to be out doing meaningful stuff with their families and friends.

I guess my point is that we would all probably be much healthier - and much happier and fulfilled - if we replaced some of the hours we spend mindlessly in front of the TV with some engaging, calorie-burning activities. Cutting the cable could be the craziest thing you ever did, which may be why it is time to actually do it.

Today ask yourself, "How would my life improve if I dropped Cable or Netflix?"

- David

CHAPTER 14

REST UP

I arise from dreams of thee
In the first sweet sleep of the night,
When the winds are breathing low,
And the stars are shining bright...

> - Percy Bysshe Shelley, "The Indian Serenade"

Romantic Poet Shelley was likely speaking of sleep in the context of true love, but his words about the "first sweet sleep of the night" almost make me want to fall asleep and rest up right now. Perhaps a little "sweet sleep" would benefit all of us, especially those who want to lose weight. Read on to see what I am talking about to see why "rest up" is good weight loss advice.

Studies show that getting a good night's sleep not only eases early morning crankiness, but helps us lose weight (7). The bad news is that Americans are pretty much sleep deprived, perhaps having as our anthem the Fifth Dimension classic "Last Night I Didn't Get to Sleep at All." In 1900, Americans slept an average of nine hours a night, and in 1970, seven hours a night. However, today it is believed to be about 6.1 hours. That is right, Americans barely get over six hours of sleep a night. In other words, if you live in America, most of your friends and family, and maybe even you, are sleep-deprived.

Why are we sleeping less? It is easy for me to think of plenty of reasons, because it almost seems like our modern lifestyle allows no time for sleep. We are just so "busy." Sleep takes a back seat to long hours at the office, soccer practices, piano recitals, meetings, television, the Internet, and so forth.

Some people have so much stress in their life, they have trouble even falling sleep. Despite the words of certain braggarts you may remember from college ("I don't need sleep!"), getting a good night's sleep is important to maintaining a healthy life, and a healthy weight. In fact recent research suggests that even sleeping in a room in which a street light shines in might increase your risk of cancer (8).

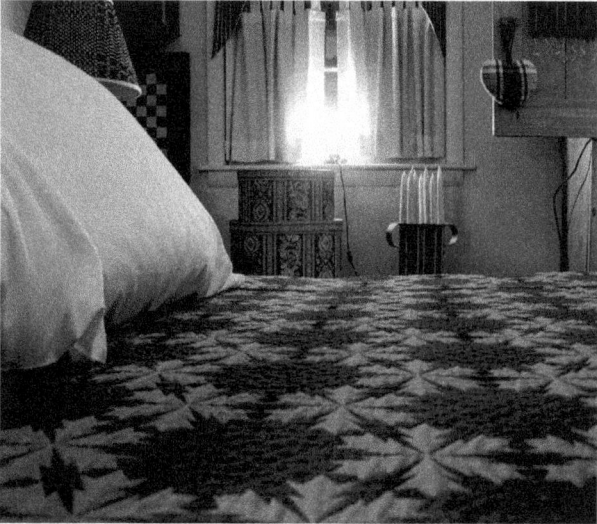

Let's examine the weight loss consequences of sleep deprivation (not even considering other problems associated with it). According to *Flip the Switch* by Dr. Robert Cooper:

- When scientists tracked 500 adults over 13 years, those who gained the most fat also had lost the most sleep.

- A study from Columbia University found that the rate of obesity is 23% higher among those who get six hours of sleep a night compared with those who average seven to eight hours.

- Sleep deprived people tend to increase their calorie consumption by 10 to 15 percent per day, compared to normal-rested individuals (9).

The same holds true for obese children. According to *Super-Sized Kids*:

- One study found that children of all ages, on average, are getting two hours less sleep per night than they are supposed to, which is nine hours per night.

- A large Japanese study of 6 and 7 year olds found a "significant connection" between late bedtime or short sleeping time, and childhood obesity.

- A large German study of 5 and 6 year olds found the same connection: less sleep means heavier kids (6).

So how do we get sleep? Dr. Cooper recommends reducing stress, sleeping in a comfortable bed, sleeping in a totally dark room, avoiding exercise right before bed, and getting up at the same time every morning, among other ideas.

Caffeine remains in the body for a significant time frame, so avoiding caffeine after 3:00 PM is probably a good idea if you want good sleep.

I have found the supplement Melatonin, cheaply available online and in a variety of stores, to be helpful. Melatonin is the hormone the body makes when we are in dark environments, so if you don't want to pop a pill, get a sleep mask, or else make your bedroom completely dark by installing black-out curtains.

Melatonin has reduced the time it takes me to get to sleep significantly. However, be aware that the long term safety of any amount of Melatonin is unknown.

So, while you have probably heard weight loss gurus tell you to "get active," an equally effective idea is to "get to sleep!"

Today evaluate your level of sleep, and whether sleep is a priority in your life. And...get some sleep tonight!

- David

Chapter 15

Get Counting (Your Steps)

At my old school, when I had a pedometer that I wore on my belt, new students usually asked me, "what is that black box on your belt?" This served as an opportunity for me to explain to them what a pedometer was.

They often followed up with the question, "why do you need a pedometer?" I usually told them it is because I liked to be active and get a lot of exercise, and the pedometer helped me do this.

By the middle of the year, the kids would always ask me how many steps I had gotten at that point in the day. It really was a kind of conversational piece, but for the serious dieter, it is an essential aid in weight loss.

For those of you who might not know what it is, a pedometer measures the number of steps a person takes in a day. More expensive ones also calculate mileage and calories burned, based on parameters you program into it. Pedometers are a nice way to keep track of your daily activity level. I think every dieter should get one, at the least to accurately know how many - or how few - steps you are getting in a day.

The popular fitness bracelets, like FitBit and Jawbone Up, act as pedometers (among other things), and allow you to connect to your smart phone. They not only measure steps, but other metrics like sleep patterns. The apps that go along with them allow you to track your calories and compete with other users to see who can get the most steps.

Experts recommend getting at least 10,000 steps a day for weight loss and weight maintenance. Based on my stride, that's walking about 4.5 miles a day. I have heard some claim that if you reach this 10,000 number, you will certainly lose weight. While I don't believe this is always true (because some people make up for the extra activity by eating more), 10,000 is a good goal.

Personally, I try to get at least 10,000 steps a day, every day, not including intense aerobic exercise. The reason I don't count my aerobic exercise in my steps is that I want aerobic exercise to be kind of like "extra credit."

The most steps I ever took was around 22,000-24,000, when I visited Washington D.C. with junior high students. I walked over 10 miles that day, if I recall correctly. I was on the move constantly. However, nothing could beat teaching kindergarten, which I taught as a substitute teacher frequently in 2005. I regularly took 12,000-14,000 steps on these days, before even leaving work. You sure have to move a lot to keep up with the young kids!

Refer back to Chapter Three for some tips on how to get more steps. Using a pedometer will force you to get creative with your movement. You'll be surprised how many creative ways you'll come up with to increase your steps.

In conclusion, wearing a pedometer gives you precise control over your activity level, and allows you to gauge whether or not you need to be more active on a particular day. Additionally, wearing a pedometer may shine the light on just how inactive you may be during the average day, acting as a motivation to move more!

Today get a device to count your steps, and try to increase that number each day.

- David

CHAPTER 16

DRINK WATER

It is important when losing weight to drink water. Water is an ancient symbol of life, nourishment, and regeneration, which is why Christians use water in the sacrament of baptism. It is no wonder water is such a powerful symbol: the human body is 60 percent water, and without water, we would die in a matter of days. To drink water is to survive and thrive.

According to *Flip the Switch*, most of us are chronically dehydrated. Our bodies naturally lose about ten cups of water a day, and this doesn't include water lost from intense exercise, and the dehydrating effects of stress, coffee, cola, and other

factors. So it seems that most of us don't drink water
to the extent we need to (9).

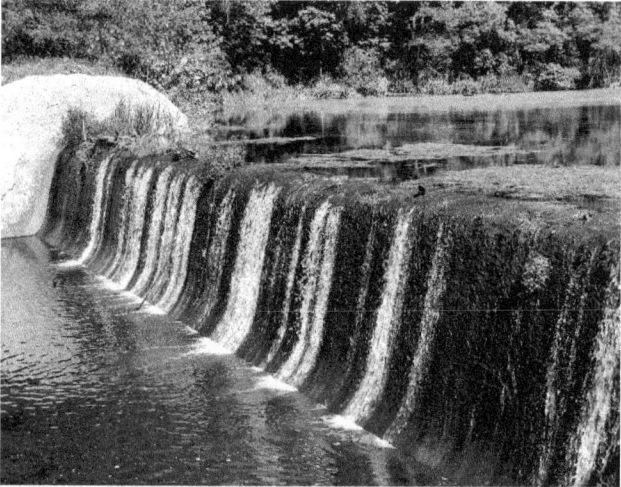

Not only are we chronically dehydrated, but our
dehydration is making it harder for us to lose weight.
Again, the research presented in *Flip the Switch* is very
telling:

- Dehydration may cause the build-up of fat
deposits, and increased fluid intake enhances the
biochemical processes that help the body release fatty
acids from fat cells in the blood stream. The message?
More water equals fewer fat deposits.

- When our bodies are dehydrated, we may
perceive dehydration signals as hunger pangs, and
eat more, so staying hydrated may help us eat less.

- A German study found that sipping two liters of water a day increased calorie burning by 100 calories. In the course of a year, with everything else equal, that will result in a loss of ten pounds (9).

- One study found that after sipping seventeen ounces of ice water, a person's metabolism is raised by thirty percent for around ninety minutes. Apparently, the body has to use extra energy to warm the water to body temperature. Drinking seventeen ounces of water seems to be especially helpful in boosting metabolism if the ice water is consumed in the morning (10).

A 2015 study found that drinking just sixteen ounces (two glasses) of water before a meal can have pretty significant weight loss effects. In the study, those who "pre-loaded" each meal with a pint of water lost 9.48 pounds over the course of the twelve week study, while those who only drank the pint before one meal, or not at all, only lost 1.76 pounds (11). The lesson? Drink a pint of water before every meal!

I try to drink a lot of water throughout the day, beginning in the morning. It keeps me hydrated and my stomach full all day. I am fortunate that our school has a water cooler. I take a big forty-four ounce cup and fill it and drink it throughout the day.

I also drink seventeen ounces or more of ice water first thing in the morning, as mentioned above. I just fill up the water bottle the night before, and put it in the fridge. By morning it is very cold, although I admit that doing this is much easier in the summer than in the winter!

It really makes sense to drink a lot of water in the morning. Would we ever go eight hours straight without any liquid? Well, that is what we do at night, so it is logical that in the morning we would need to seriously rehydrate ourselves!

In conclusion, consuming enough water is an important component of any good weight loss plan. It is pretty cheap too: get a big cup, go to a faucet, and proceed to drink.

Today commit to drink more water. Buy a big (but also convenient) water bottle and take it to work with you.

- David

CHAPTER 17

SET GOALS (AND REMIND YOURSELF OF THEM)

If weight loss was easy, we'd all be thin. It was easy for ancient man to stay at a normal weight, because he didn't know where his next meal was coming from, and would burn plenty of calories tackling and killing prehistoric animals.

It is important to set goals! Not so long ago, you had to burn a lot of calories just to get calories, and this is still true in many parts of the world. Today, we still have our instinctual love of rich, fatty foods, but we aren't nearly as active, so we have to use our ration and reason (our minds) to overcome our natural love of high-calorie foods, and inactivity.

This is where goal-setting come in. I find that it is helpful to set goals, and devise a clear and realistic time frame to achieve the set goals. Also, I make it a point to constantly reminding myself of the goal. I tend to do it like this:

General Goal: Lose fat, gain muscle

Reasons for Goal: Look thinner and in better shape by the summer

Ways to Achieve Goal: Weight lift every other day; run every other day; walk on non-running days

This example is broad, but you get the idea. After setting these goals, I find ways to remind myself of them. I write them on a card in my wallet, post them on my fridge, or, send myself an email reminder every day!

Another thing I used to do was visualize myself reaching some sort of goal at the end of a segment of exercise, in order to motivate me to get through the exercise. If you are not following me, let me explain. I used this some in high school (this example is very "high school," so be warned).

For example, if I was getting ready to ask a particular girl out, but wanted to lose a little weight first, I would make a game out of the sprints. After the first sprint, it would be like I walked up to her, the second, starting a conversation, and so forth, until I visualized going on a date (nothing beyond this, so get your mind out of the gutter!).

Sure, this is a high school male example, but you get my drift. It was a vivid reminder of my goals, and why I was out there dying in the hot sun. It made the hot sun beating down upon the track, and upon me, more bearable. In fact, I still have fond memories of nearly dying out there!

You need not look at goals quite like this, but I think finding ways to keep your goals (and the reasons) on your mind constantly is essential to losing weight. There is a verse in the Bible about shining light in the darkness, and the darkness not mastering it.

Shining light on something exposes it for what it is. Continually keeping your goals in your mind is like constantly shining light on your overeating and inactivity, exposing them as empty and contrary to what you want to be.

Some people find that posting a "fat photo" of themselves helps them keep their goals, while others prefer displaying a thin photo from the past.

Sometimes a photo of the grandkids is what it takes. I find that being healthy is like anything else, which is to say that if you value it highly enough, you will make an effort to do it.

Take a few minutes to ask yourself why you are losing weight and getting healthy, or why you want to keep the weight off? Write down your goals so you can always keep them (and the outcome) in your mind.

Today set some goals and make sure they are available and in front of you when you need to remember them!

- David

CHAPTER 18

SUBSTITUTE

There are a variety of low and lower calorie foods available these days, like fat-free sour cream, light butter, and sugar-free ice cream. Most are marketed toward dieters and health enthusiasts. I have even seen *calorie-free* foods available! Personally, if there is a lighter option, I tend to eat it, unless the light option is not really worth the price (since light options sometimes are more expensive).

Also, I tend to choose lower calorie options, but not necessarily completely fat-free options, because I know the importance of good fats in my diet. As those who struggle with their weight know, calories add up very quickly, and saving a few calories here and there helps in the long run.

Below I compare calorie values of some light and regular calorie foods, so you can see that in the course of a day, choosing a lighter option over a full-calorie version really makes a difference. If you are not looking into lighter versions of your favorite high-calorie foods, you are ignoring an easy way to lose some weight. The calorie values and serving size are listed below, with the calorie savings in **bold**.

Regular Butter: 100 (tbsp)
Whipped Butter: 67 (tbsp) **-37**

Regular Wheat Bread: 90 (slice)
Light Bread: 35 (slice) **-55**

Regular Cheese - 100 (1/4 c)
Part-Skim Mozzarella Cheese 80 (1/4 c) **-20**

2% Milk 120 (c)
Skim Milk 80 (c) **-40**

Regular Non-Fat Yogurt 120 (6 oz)
Light Yogurt 80 (6 oz) **-40**

Ground Beef 313 (4 oz)
Ground Turkey 170 (4 oz) **-143**

Regular Pasta 210 (2 oz dry)
"Creamette 150" Pasta 150 (2 oz dry) **-60**

Regular Cola 150 (12 oz)
Diet Soft Drink 0 (12 oz) **-150**

While unrealistic, if you substitute all of these in a day, you would save 545 calories. This amounts to 3815 calories in a week.

At this rate, you would lose a little over a pound of fat a week, all things equal, just by making these few substitutions.

In addition to lowering your calories, by making these choices, you would increase your fiber and consume less sugar and trans-fats! I have found that eating lighter versions of foods takes a little getting used to, but only a little.

I avoid foods that are *radically* lower in fat and calories than the original, because sometimes these do not taste very good, and can be expensive. Also, some studies have shown that sugar-free and low-fat foods don't really help people lose weight, because they give us a taste for the real thing, so we eat more to compensate.

Bear this in mind when consuming light foods. Finding lighter options is usually pretty easy, since they are often available beside the regular options at the supermarket.

One example of how I substitute is the way that I make pumpkin muffins. By using applesauce instead of the 3/4 cup of oil, I save over *1200* calories!

I have used sucralose (Splenda) as well, but I am not necessarily convinced of the long-term safety of it, so I have cut down on that particular substitution.

Often you can search online to find healthy substitutions that you can use in recipes! So, with the wide variety of light foods available, and plenty of light recipes available, get started substituting!!

Today explore lighter options at the grocery store and in restaurants.

- David

CHAPTER 19

GO WITH FEELING GOOD

As we lose weight, we look and feel better, and get excited. This effect is noticeable almost immediately. However, food and inactivity are strong addictions, and negative influences in our lives, and sometimes when we reach a plateau, or go through a stressful period in life, we shelve our good efforts, and revert back to depending on things like sugar and fat to feel good.

There is much more long-term satisfaction in living a disciplined life than there is in the short-term satisfaction that we get from gorging or being inactive. Of course, being disciplined is easier said than done, especially when you have just gotten home from a stressful day at work and potato chips are calling your name!

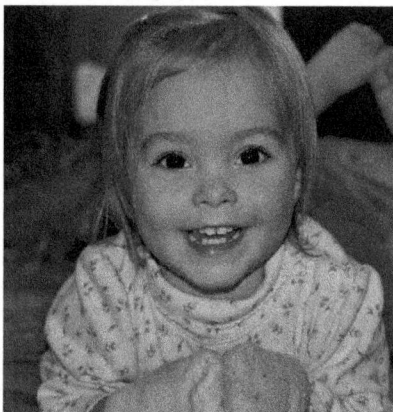

In this chapter, I am suggesting that we need to tap into the good things that are happening in our lives because of being healthy, and focus on them all the time. In other words, we need to be optimistic! Losing weight - and keeping it off - is a struggle, but there are very tangible rewards that result from even slight weight loss.

I think we need to "go with feeling good," that is, remind ourselves how good we feel and look from our weight loss. I can think of four examples of how I tried to put this into action, and I hope my experiences give you some ideas.

In the fall of 2008, I was the chaperone for my school's homecoming dance. It was catered by a local Italian place, and I ate a good bit, mainly because I had run five miles and lifted for forty minutes a few hours earlier, and I needed the calories (especially the protein). However, when I was tempted to eat handfuls of potato chips later in the night, I remembered how good I had been feeling lately since I had lost weight.

I also looked around at dancing students, and thought about much it meant to me that at thirty I was in good enough shape to keep up with them on the basketball court when I played afterschool with them. I also thought about how I was in better shape at thirty than when I attended my own homecoming dance! I was grateful for where I was, and that alone was enough for me to forgo a bunch of chips (I did eat a few). Looking back, I should have quietly said to myself how grateful I was to be at this point.

Another example happened a few days later. My wife and I were walking around our neighborhood after church, and I remarked how nice it was outside, and how great it was that we were able to walk, and how I enjoyed being in shape. It wasn't a huge revelation, but I was grateful for something as simple as being in shape enough to enjoy the great weather.

What does it hurt to focus on what we have accomplished? It doesn't hurt, and in fact, it should be a tool to keep us on the path of health and wellness. It is very important to speak positive thoughts out loud.

In early 2009, I went to the doctor. The nurse took my pulse, and when she read "48," she said "that can't be right" and took it again. Again, it was "48." She asked, "Do you exercise a lot or something?" I said "yes." The doctor asked the same thing, and told me to keep up the good work.

A 48 pulse is very healthy and in the "athlete" range. This made me feel really good! I told my wife, my friends, and am writing about it here, not to brag, but to keep it in my mind so I will always remember the benefits of health, especially on days I may be tempted to get instant gratification from gorging.

Finally, I get mistaken for being a lot younger, and this happens a lot. My students will even fight with me about my age. A few days ago a student and I got into a discussion about something related to age. I mentioned I was 37. She said no way was that possible and accused me of joking with her. When I insisted it was true, she argued with me. I remember these examples whenever I feel like skipping running or wanting to overeat.

How can you "go with feeling good?" I suggest reminding yourself of the benefits frequently. Start a weight-loss blog or write something every day on your calendar that reminds you why it is a great to eat right or exercise. For example, you may write on Monday's agenda "I look better in a swimsuit." Every time you check your daily calendar, that will be fresh in your mind. Get creative! It is your life!

The best way to think about weight loss is to focus on the long haul. We can't recapture our youth, nor should we obsess about something impossible, but we can improve the way we feel now and in the future. If we are healthy, and stay healthy, we know we are doing our part to look and feel better in the future, i.e. we are going with feeling good!

Today think of the positive benefits you're experiencing because of your weight loss program. Focus on these and feel good!

- David

Chapter 20

Think Young

When I was growing up, I thought that when people got past a certain age (around 28ish), they had kids, gained weight, and started looking and thinking old. Instead, I choose to think young!

I suppose if you *think* aging happens like this, then it *will* happen this way. If you think you will turn into an old, overweight, person at 28, you probably will be an old, overweight, 28-year old!

However, I don't think that aging dooms us to weight gain, or looking and feeling old. As I get older, I notice that a lot of people my age (37 as of now) look old, and some look young. Some are healthy, some are not.

Reputable scientists tell us that it makes sense to think young, because a person's chronological age, and his or her "real" age, are two different things. There are plenty of 30-somethings that are "younger" than many 20-somethings, based on overall health and lifestyle choices. A 21-year old obese smoker is probably "older" than a fit, non-smoking 30-year old with good genetics.

This means that with a few lifestyle changes, you can basically "grow younger" in a matter of months. This is a strong motivation for me to lose weight, and keep it off, because I want to be active and healthy for a long time.

I find it extremely sad when a person is unable to live a full life because of lifestyle choices. I have had relatives who lost quality of life, and eventually passed away young, because of obesity.

My uncle was morbidly obese as long as I knew him, and I have fond memories eating at his family's home on Christmas Eve. I also recall the 2-inch layer of butter in the bottom of the macaroni he made! Sadly, he died too young of a heart attack. He was also suffering from diabetic complications before his death. He was in his forties and could barely walk as gangrene overtook his legs.

Surveys of really old people (in their 90s and 100s) show that they think young. They try to keep up with the latest technology and ideas. In other words, they don't resign themselves to being old and "out-of-it." I think this is the key to thinking, and thus being, young. Staying involved, and being active, is going to help us feel young, and, if we are active, stay fit. I can think of three great examples.

The first example is a professor I had in college. He was in his 80s when I was in his class. He was teaching a full schedule, and was still running marathons, which means he was probably more active than most of the students on campus! He attended my brother's wedding in 2007, in good health. He once told me that his secret was drinking Retsina, a Greek white wine! I don't know about that, but he embodies youthful thinking.

Second, I think of a friend of my grandma's named Bob. In 1994, Bob was diagnosed with prostate cancer. I loaned him a few alternative medicine books related to cancer (I was 15 at the time). Bob improved his diet, became more active, and continued working hard on his farm. He is alive and kicking today, and cancer free.

Finally, the last example is my mom. She has always eaten well, exercised, and taken care of herself. A few days ago I was visiting my grandma, and our cousin was there as well. I hadn't met this cousin before and we started talking about the past. I found out my cousin was 70. My mom is 65. The difference between them was night and day. My mom was active in the conversation and looked youthful. Our cousin not only looked like she was almost 80, but she asked the same question three times.

The best (and original) website dedicated to this principle of a true age is RealAge.Com. Visit the site and take the real age test, and see what your "real age" is. If it is not as young as you like, make lifestyle changes, and check back later. I tend to come in about ten years younger than I am. I have signed up for their emails, and they are contain valuable information.

Let me briefly state that I think obsessing with looking younger can be unhealthy. Aging is a normal part of human life, and cannot be erased with drugs, vitamins, or plastic surgery. While I try to cultivate a healthy lifestyle, and work to look and feel young, obsessing over it is not a good idea.

Also, I think we must examine our motivations for trying to be young. Looking and feeling young should not be about recapturing lost youth (the past is the past), returning to a moment from our youth, or "being eighteen again." It is good to be grown-up, and trying to be young should not be an excuse to act like a teenager.

In conclusion, working to look and feel young is a strong motivator to get healthy. I enjoy going to reunions and other events, and having my peers say "man, you look like you haven't aged a bit!" That could be because I am in better shape now than when I was in high school. Think young. Get healthy. Be young.

Today start thinking young! There is no reason to resign yourself to "acting old."

- David

CHAPTER 21

WEIGH AND MEASURE

Weight loss experts tell us that Americans eat portion sizes that are way too big, and we also consistently underestimate how much we actually eat, which is why we need to weigh and measure. Say it with me: *weigh and measure*!

Some people underestimate their energy intake significantly (12)! This may explain why so many Americans say, "I have tried to lose weight, but it just won't work!" and then they blame their thyroid, metabolism, or genetics for their obesity.

The reality is that what they did was *think* they were making changes, but they were really improperly estimating their calorie intake.

The solution I have found to this problem, besides keeping a food log, is to measure almost everything I eat.

Sometimes I do estimate, especially with lower calorie foods, but since I measure the majority of the time, I am able to estimate more accurately. My friends and family probably get annoyed that I am always measuring out portions, although I don't (yet) carry measuring tools with me!

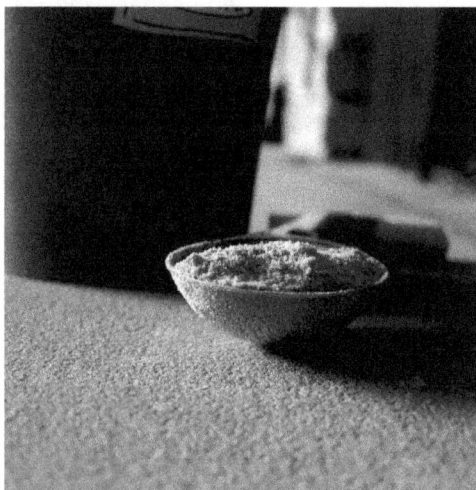

To do this on a regular basis, you will need basic measuring tools. These include measuring spoons, liquid and solid cup measures, and a food scale of some kind.

Generally these tools are inexpensive, and easy-to-find. I suggest investing in a fairly nice digital scale, which can weigh in ounces and grams. I bought one for about $15.00 on sale, and it came with a plastic bowl.

Of course, with some foods, like snack foods and crackers, it may be easier just to count the items you eat, rather than weigh them out. However, whether you are weighing or just portioning items, it is key to keep track of what you are eating!

Let me give you an example of a typical meal I eat, and how I measure the contents. Last night's dinner was cheesy potato tots with homemade ketchup.

I weighed out the potato tots to get sixteen ounces. Then I weighed the cheese, and finally measured out the ketchup using cup measurers.

Another night, I had turkey burgers on low-calorie bread rounds, peas, and some pistachio nuts.

The turkey burgers and bread rounds are pre-made, so there is no need to measure them; I know they contain 140 calories per burger and 90 calories per round.

I measured out the peas using a cup measurer. I count the number of pistachio nuts. This may seem like a lot of effort, but it really isn't, especially since it is now a habit. Plus, there is a powerful benefit: at the end of the day, I know what I have eaten, and very few hidden calories have sneaked into my body!

Another tip I have is to keep recipes pretty consistent. By the time you "add some oil here," and "throw in some extra cheese there," your well-measured, light recipe, has a bunch of added, and hidden, calories.

Measuring before cooking is just as important as measuring afterwards. I know some cooks who will take a light recipe and "enhance" it so much that is isn't light after they get done with it!

Measuring may be a little trickier when you eat somewhere other than your house. As I mentioned above, the more you measure, the better you will become at estimating food portions and calories.

Another problem is that your homemade recipe for a certain dish (like spaghetti) may be much healthier than the recipe prepared by the cook at work or your friends. You should keep this in mind when estimating calories.

Overall, measuring and weighing food on a daily basis can save you hundreds of calories a day, by eliminating hidden calories, and encouraging portion control.

Today invest in some food measuring tools, or if you have them already, dust them off.

- David

CHAPTER 22

EAT EGGS FOR BREAKFAST

This may be the strangest tip yet. You may wonder why in the world I am telling you what to eat for breakfast. Well, give me a minute! It will all make sense soon.

Eggs have gotten a bad rap over the years, so much that people might even be surprised that I would suggest it is good to eat eggs for breakfast. What was once considered a wholesome, high-protein food, became a nutritional pariah.

Let me defend eggs for a minute. In the rush to condemn anything with fat or cholesterol in the 1970s and 1980s, it was in vogue to trash eggs.

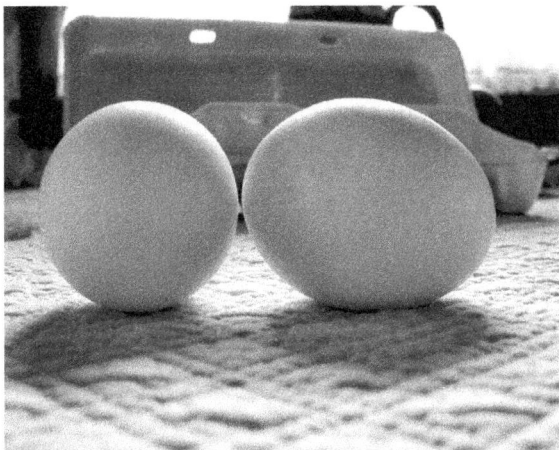

Yes, eggs contain cholesterol, but experts aren't even sure that cholesterol from foods has an effect on blood cholesterol, or that blood cholesterol is even correlated with heart attacks!

In fact emerging research suggests cholesterol isn't even a major factor in heart disease (13).

Personally, I eat eggs a lot, and my cholesterol levels are perfect. Of course, my one example doesn't prove or disprove anything about the relationship of eggs and cholesterol, but I do eat eggs at many meals.

I may be onto something actually. A 2008 study suggested that eating eggs for breakfast may help you lose weight.

DAVID AND JONATHAN BENNETT

In that study of dieters, those who ate two scrambled eggs and unbuttered toast (with jelly) for breakfast lost **65 percent more weight** than those that had a bagel and cream cheese for breakfast. They also reported higher energy levels than those who ate the bagel breakfast (14).

I am sure that a lot of people would assume that the bagel and cream cheese would have been healthier, and provide more energy, but this study shows that those who had eggs and toast lost significantly more weight than the bagel group.

Another study looked at adolescent girls and their breakfast habits. Those who ate a high protein breakfast of either eggs or lean meat (as opposed to cereal) felt more full throughout the day, and snacked less in the evening. Their brain activity even reflected the increased fullness (15).

Apparently, the protein in eggs helps people feel more full, and this feeling lasts for quite a while after eating the eggs themselves.

However, we must remember that every participant in the first study also restricted their calories.

Sadly, this means that we can't fry up a big sausage, bacon, and cheese omelet every morning and expect to lose weight. Eggs for breakfast may be part of a weight-loss plan, but they aren't magical diet bullets!

There is a financial benefit to eggs too: they are usually cheap. They are pretty high right now thanks to a bird flu epidemic but overall the price of a dozen eggs is very reasonable.

Today fry up a few eggs for breakfast and skip the cereal or toast, and see what happens!

- David

CHAPTER 23

EAT THE RIGHT FAT

Fat is bad. If you wish to lose weight, you must avoid fat, right? Wrong.

This myth may be hurting your weight loss efforts! Your body needs some fat in order to function properly. It is true that Americans eat way too much fat, but the main problem seems to be that Americans eat too much of *everything*, including the *wrong types* of fat.

Specifically, it seems that Americans eat too much trans-fat, saturated fat, and Omega-6 fats, and too little monounsaturated fats and omega-3 fats. In this chapter, I will focus on monounsaturated fats, also known as Omega-9 fats.

Monounsaturated fats are liquid at room temperature, but solidify when refrigerated. They are present in olive oil, peanuts, almonds, macadamia nuts, avocados, and other foods.

Technically they are not essential, but they are beneficial when consumed in normal amounts. Like other fats, monounsaturated fats are energy dense, containing nine calories per gram. Some new research suggests that monounsaturated fats may help us lose body fat, specifically harmful belly fat, which I will address in a moment.

You may be inclined to think that body fat is body fat, but fat stored around the stomach and other internal organs, called visceral fat, is more dangerous to the body than fat stored near the hips. Belly fat (a "beer gut," or "spare tire") is associated with inflammation in the body, and puts you at risk of heart disease, high blood pressure, diabetes, and other diseases.

Thus, when losing weight, losing belly fat is important, if you wish to see a health improvement result from your weight loss efforts.

Okay, okay, now to my point. Research suggests that a diet high in monounsaturated fats may help you lose weight, specifically belly fat, more easily. In a 2007 study, participants placed on a high monounsaturated fat diet lost weight (and belly fat) without adding extra exercise to their routines, or restricting calories (16).

This suggests that monounsaturated fats may have an important role in maintaining a healthy weight. It also may mean that dieting will be easier if you are consuming enough of these good fats.

Nuts are high in monounsaturated fats, as are peanuts (not a true nut). Snacking on these items will help you increase your intake of Omega-9 fats. Also, since olive oil is high in monounsaturated fats, cooking with olive oil is recommended.

On days when I am low in monounsaturated fats, I have even eaten a teaspoon of pure olive oil before bed. A diet tracking program, like My Fitness Pal, will help you see if you are getting enough monounsaturated fats in your diet.

Before I end, let me say that I consume a good number of monounsaturated fats each day, and believe I am healthier for it. I buy peanuts in the shell, and snack on them whenever I am hungry, which increases the amount of monounsaturated fat in my diet.

However, remember that monounsaturated fats still contain calories. If you are trying to lose weight, you don't want to go overboard on any food, even if it is good for you. So in conclusion, consuming more monounsaturated fat may make your weight loss efforts easier, and get rid of that pesky - and dangerous - beer gut.

Buy some olive oil and stock up on some nuts. They make a great and filling snack.

- David

CHAPTER 24

MAKE IT HOMEMADE AND LIGHTER

I became fed up with buying ketchup in the store a few months ago. I didn't like consuming all that high fructose corn syrup. I also wasn't too happy paying nearly double that price for lower carb ketchup. Then I looked at the ingredients on the bottle: tomato paste, water, and vinegar. I am hardly a chef, but that didn't seem too complicated to make.

So I started looking for some recipes online. What I found was amazing. There are hundreds of recipes for ketchup, just waiting for me to modify them based on my own tastes and calorie needs. The ketchup I was buying in the store contains 20 calories per tablespoon, along with 5 grams of carbs. My homemade ketchup (recipe below!) contains **7** calories, and **1** carb per tablespoon.

This might not seem like a huge deal, but over the course of a week, that saves me quite a few calories, and money. There are many recipes online for pretty much everything you can think of. I went looking for a wheat-free pizza crust. Sure enough, I found one whose crust consists of flax meal, parmesan cheese, and eggs.

I previously used a whole wheat pizza recipe. The whole wheat recipe had 12 "net" carbs per slice versus **1** "net" carbs per slice in the flax recipe. A "net" carb is the total carbs minus the fiber content, since fiber calories aren't used by the body. I'll admit that when I first started looking for a low carb pizza crust recipe I thought even the Internet would be unable to complete that task. I was wrong. I'm glad I was.

I will list the ketchup recipe below, but all you have to do is go to a search engine and look for "low carb," "low fat," "gluten free," "reduced calorie," or "light" versions of your favorite recipes, depending on your needs.

I never imagined flax, parmesan cheese, and eggs could make a pizza crust until I started searching. I didn't know that you could substitute applesauce for oil in muffins. Guess what? You won't know that there are healthier versions of your favorite foods unless you search them out, and make them at home. Even if you aren't much of a chef, you can still make your food healthier by seeking out recipes that suit your diet needs.

Below is my homemade ketchup recipe. It is very easy to make, and cheap.

2, six ounce cans of tomato paste

3/4 cup water

3/4 cup white vinegar

1 tsp onion powder

1 tsp salt substitute (Morton's Lite Salt)

1/4 tsp black pepper

1/4 teaspoon cinnamon

1 tsp mustard powder

1 tsp coriander

Stevia to taste

Blend all the ingredients. To make it tangier, add more vinegar relative to water. To make it less tangy, increase the amount of water to vinegar. To thicken it, reduce the vinegar and water. To thin it out, add more vinegar and/or water. This makes about 1.5 cups of ketchup. Nutritionally, per tablespoon, it contains:

Calories – 7
Fat – 0 g
Carbohydrate – 1 g
Protein – 1 g
Sodium – 55 mg
Potassium – 133 mg
Vitamin A – 108 IU
Vitamin C – 2 mg

Today get creative and look up some homemade and light versions of your favorite foods!

- David

CHAPTER 25

I Don't Believe In Weight Loss Supplements, But If I Did, I'd Believe In This

I usually joke that if a chemical causes you to lose weight, we have a name for that: a poison!

For years, people have been searching for a magical weight loss supplement that allows you to eat everything you want and not gain fat. As the title of this post indicates, I don't really believe such a supplement exists. However, there is one that may actually not only cause you to lose fat, but also help you gain muscle. And, the good news, is that it is dirt cheap.

What am I talking about? The chemical's name is betaine (pronounced BEET-uh-een), also known as trimethylglycine or TMG. It naturally occurs in beets, spinach, and quinoa. It is available in anhydrous form (pure betaine) or bound to hydrochloride as betaine hydrochloride. The latter form is sometimes promoted to improve digestion.

A variety of recent studies suggest betaine may help people burn fat while gaining muscle. The most exciting research was recently performed at the College of Springfield in Massachusetts.

Researchers had a group of males weight-train for six weeks. One group took 1,250 milligrams of betaine twice a day, and the control group (which was also weight training) took a placebo. The researchers reported that the subjects taking betaine **increased muscle mass by four pounds** and **arm size by ten percent (!)**, while experiencing a **decrease in body fat of seven percent**. The placebo group experienced none of these effects (17).

Wow! While the study was small, and certainly is preliminary, I can't help but be excited by betaine. I have taken it for years in the HCL form, and recently, based on this study, I have upped my intake closer to what was given in the study. Luckily betaine is cheap.

While my anecdote which follows is hardly proof of anything, I'll still share. Since taking extra betaine, combined with running, Tabata, the Insanity and Asylum workout programs (which build muscle), I have noticed that I've gained about eight pounds. Sounds bad right? Well, here is the interesting thing.

The shirts and pants that I bought when I was eight pounds lighter still fit perfectly. In other words, I don't seem to have gained any fat during this period, but my muscles are noticeably bigger. I do seem to be experiencing the fat loss and muscle gain after upping my betaine intake.

So, while recognizing that the research is preliminary, I am pretty excited about the possibilities of betaine.

Today look into getting some betaine. Trying betaine can't hurt, right?

- David

CHAPTER 26

A MILE A MINUTE?

What if I told you there was a type of workout that can burn as many calories in four minutes as you would in an hour of running (18)? You might think I'm crazy and promoting some nutty fad. I promise you, this book is not about fads that don't work and cost a fortune.

Well, there is such a workout that can, at least based on preliminary research, burn a lot of calories from a brief period of exercise, and it is called Tabata. It is a specific type of interval training.

It sounds exotic, but it is just named after the Japanese researcher who pioneered it, Izumi Tabata.

The good news is that it may actually work. The bad news? Well, it isn't exactly four minutes of a stroll through the park. It is four minutes of absolute hell unleashed on your body.

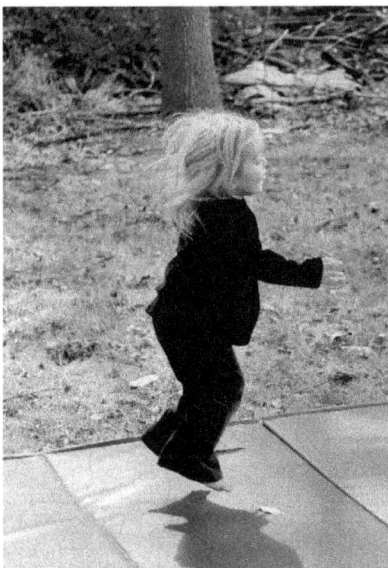

In his studies, Tabata's program burned a massive number of calories during and after the exercise (due to its intensity, the ramped up metabolic effects may last as much as 12 hours afterwards), as well as increasing overall aerobic (oxygen processing) and anaerobic (strength) capacity (19).

So, unlike other workouts, if done properly, Tabata seems to increase your heart, lung, and muscle health all at once.

Tabata starts with a ten minute light warm-up, followed by intense exercises for twenty seconds, resting for ten seconds, and then repeating this 20 seconds on, 10 seconds off, protocol for four minutes.

For Tabata to work, you must work out extremely intensely. In other words, for each of those twenty second bursts, you have to give your all, to the point that you should be out of breath by the end of that brief period. If you can "recover" significantly during the ten second rest, you aren't doing Tabata properly.

So here it is segmented for those who need to see it explained that way:

Exercise 1: 20 seconds on, 10 second break, 20 seconds on, 10 second break

Exercise 2: 20 seconds on, 10 second break, 20 seconds on, 10 second break

Exercise 3: 20 seconds on, 10 second break, 20 seconds on, 10 second break

Exercise 4: 20 seconds on, 10 second break, 20 seconds on, you're done! (finally)

There are a variety of exercises you can use. I prefer ones that are explosive in their movements,

DAVID AND JONATHAN BENNETT

and that engage a variety of muscle groups at once, because this makes for a more intense workout.

Exercises like squat jumps (jumping high and landing in a squat), burpees, moving push-ups (doing a push-up, moving to the left, doing a push-up, moving back, and so forth), hurdle jumping, etc. are examples.

You can do Tabata with more traditional exercises like jumping jacks too, but make it intense.

I like Tabata because it is over so quickly. I can usually get motivated to do a four minute workout. I also like that I can do it anywhere.

I have to lessen the intensity when I am in my work clothes, but I can still do something for four minutes anywhere I am.

I will often do "static hold" Tabata throughout the day. I know this won't burn as many calories as an intense one, but it builds muscle. For example, I will hold the squat and lunge positions. Also holding the push up position an inch off the ground can be very intense. This is much harder than it sounds, so give it a try.

There are some great mobile apps you can use to enhance your Tabata workouts. Just go to your App Store of choice and search "tabata." Many have plenty of pre-defined workouts, and some allow you to create your workout combinations from various workouts.

Today try a four minute Tabata workout from hell.

- David

CHAPTER 27

START LIKING IT ROUGH

Get your mind out of the gutter; I'm talking about fiber!

Fiber, also known as roughage, is an important part of the human diet. Fiber is technically a class of carbohydrates that humans can't digest. Because of this, fiber passes through the body undigested, and helps digestion.

Fiber comes in two forms, soluble and insoluble.

Soluble fiber will partially dissolve in water and adds bulk to your stool. Soluble fiber is found in oats, legumes, and psyllium husks (an ingredient in Metamucil). It helps normalize digestion, relieves constipation, and can make you feel full because it expands in the stomach.

Insoluble fiber doesn't dissolve in water. It has many benefits similar to soluble fiber. It is found in whole wheat and the peels of fruits and vegetables.

Fiber is technically a carbohydrate, but humans don't have the necessary enzymes to break it down. Because of this, fiber in food reduces the absorbable calories and carbohydrates in a food.

Total Carbohydrates minus fiber carbohydrates equals "net carbs." So, if a low carb tortilla has 12 grams of carbs, and has 5 grams of fiber, then the "net carbs" are 7 grams.

Labels vary as to whether the unabsorbable fiber calories are counted in the total calories or not. Apparently manufacturers don't have to include insoluble fiber in the calorie totals. So, usually the total calories already excludes the fiber calories, but in some cases fiber in a food may reduce the number of calories you see on the label.

So, are you not convinced yet?

In a recent study published in the <u>Annals Of Internal Medicine</u>, pre-diabetic individuals were either placed on a special restrictive diet, or simply told to eat thirty grams of fiber or more, with no other changes in diet or exercise. After a year, the group that ate fiber experienced the same health benefits as those who followed a special diet: weight loss and a reduction in inflammation, blood pressure, and blood sugar (20).

See why fiber is so important? It makes you feel full, helps digestion, and can increase your overall health. That is the good news. The bad news is that we don't get nearly enough.

Most people get around 15 grams of fiber per day, while the recommended amount is around 30-40 grams a day. I remember some days in college, when I was eating horribly, I would maybe get 5 grams a day.

If you are on a lower carb diet like me, you may need to add fiber supplements to your diet. Since I keep track of my food on my computer, I know my fiber intake. On low days, I add psyllium fiber from a generic version of Metamucil. I also get fiber from vegetables, nuts, fruits, and low carb bread products (which often add high fiber ingredients to reduce absorbable carbs).

So, don't be afraid to get some roughage in your diet.

Today buy some high fiber foods, and even a fiber supplement if necessary.

- David

CHAPTER 28

KEEP TRACK OF YOUR FOOD AND ACTIVITY

I am a firm believer in logging your food and activity. Not to brag (well, maybe just a little), but I have kept track of my food and exercise intake since 2007.

I have mentioned this in many of these chapters. It has benefited me immensely to have a comprehensive record of my nutrition and exercise over the last eight years.

Research is conflicting as to whether logging your food and activity increases weight loss.

Some studies say "yes," while others say it doesn't make a difference. I believe that it probably does make a difference, for those who are both committed and educated, and those willing to carefully observe their portion sizes.

The main reason I suggest you keep track of your food and activity is that it is very easy to sneak hidden calories into your day.

A 1992 study found that people often underestimate their daily calories and overestimate their activity (21).

A friend of mine did this in high school. He claimed he "only ate 1200 calories a day" and yet he was a hundred pounds overweight.

His parents frantically took him to doctors to figure out what was wrong, spending hundreds of dollars in the process.

Considering during the period he "only ate 1200 calories a day" I saw him eat an entire bag of pretzels with that many calories as a snack, I guarantee he was seriously underestimating his calories.

Logging your food and activity intake is a great way to overcome the human tendency to underestimate your intake.

I use Fitday, which is a PC program. I started using it before smart phones came around, and I am used to it, and like it.

However, there are a lot of nice apps around that make the job a lot easier, like My Fitness Pal. These apps allow you to scan a barcode and get nutrition information easily.

It is beyond the scope of this chapter to explain how these apps work.

However, I highly suggest you get one of these apps and start logging your food and activity accurately right away.

Here are a few tips to make this work for you:

- Make sure to get accurate information. Weigh, measure, count, etc., what you are eating to make sure you are recording the right amount of food.

- Record *everything*. Include your coffee (which may include calories from half and half, etc.). The little things here and there can make a difference.

- Record it as soon as possible. It is easy to forget what you ate if you don't record it quickly.

- If you can't record it right away, take a photo of your plate. I use this at buffets in particular. I take a photo of each plate, which allows me to go back later and record my food accurately.

Today explore calorie tracking apps, and play around with them. Then, actually use them!

- David

Chapter 29

Know When To Take A Break

I always emphasize to people who ask about my weight loss that for me it wasn't a diet, but a lifestyle change geared towards health, not necessarily being thin. Granted, eating healthily and working out tend to lead to thinness, but certainly not being model thin, which is often unhealthy.

Why am I mentioning this? It's because a healthy lifestyle will always have room for sweets and higher calorie foods as well as days off from exercising.

For example, denying yourself any sweet food, for your entire life, is unrealistic. What matters is that you can put the foods in perspective and eat them occasionally.

I used to go days without sweet foods and then get a hankering and binge. Then the cycle would start over.

During recent years when I finally got fit, I eat sweets, a couple of days a week in small amounts. Guess what? The binges were a thing of past and I lost weight; and I've kept it off.

So, enjoy the foods you love, just occasionally and always as a part of an overall healthy diet and fitness plan. I will use it sometimes, but I don't like the word "moderation." Some foods should not be eaten frequently, even if in moderation.

Eating moderate sized portions of unhealthy foods occasionally is my preferred method. If you truly are focused on your goal and supported by friends and family, you will be able to find a place for those treats every now and then.

The same is true for exercise. Your body needs a break, especially with strength training. In fact, over-exercising can weaken your immune system, undoing a major benefit of exercise. I tend to work out 5-6 days a week, but always take one full day off and make another day a more moderate workout. There may even be a benefit to taking a week off every so often to recover.

Today, if you have been exercising hard and/or eating right for a while, take and enjoy a break. You deserve it.

- Jonathan

CHAPTER 30

CRANK UP THE MUSIC

If you want to have a longer, more effective workout, then use a portable music device. Studies show that listening to music while exercising increases exercise times (22). I personally find that a driving beat in a musical style I enjoy can get me pumped up to not only start working out on days when I feel lazy, but also to increase my intensity and workout length.

Researchers aren't necessarily sure why music makes us able to exercise longer. Hypotheses abound. One is that the body associates music with movement, and that music encourages movement. Another is that music brings out strong emotions, which increases the intensity of exercise. Some speculate that music is simply a good distraction, and makes an arduous task like exercise more interesting.

Either way, music makes working out more enjoyable. With some mp3 players selling for as low as ten dollars, there is no excuse not to use this workout enhancer.

The best way to listen to music is to get a small player and an armband or waist clip. That way the player doesn't affect your mobility. You also have the advantage of loading a variety of music (in some cases up to thousands of songs). If your player takes batteries, get rechargeable ones since regular batteries can be expensive and the players are often drains.

What music should you have on your player? Basically whatever motivates you to workout. Some people, however, find that driving dance songs are helpful for good workouts. I find that any music that inspires me at that moment is helpful.

Today buy or dust off your MP3 player, and load it with songs to get you motivated!

- Jonathan

CHAPTER 31

MAKE YOUR WORKOUTS COUNT

I've often seen people use the fitness room at the YMCA to walk slowly on the treadmill, which I always kind of thought was a little pointless since they could just walk outside without paying for the gym. Granted, I think about this the most when people (including me) are waiting to use the booked machines!

The point? Although it's important to start off slowly and work at your level, it's also necessary to exert enough energy (depending on age and health, of course) to work up a good sweat and get out of breath.

I've read in the past that if you can sing, you're not working out hard enough. Otherwise, what really is the point of going to the gym? A recent *Time* magazine article seems to confirm this. It's called "The Myth Of Moderate Exercise" and is worth reading (23).

To see the aerobic and calorie-burning effects of exercise, you really do have to up your intensity levels. The human body evolved to benefit from regular bursts of intensity (such as running from a wild animal).

Here are a few tips to get a more intense workout.

- Play competitive sports. The more you can get into an activity, the more likely you'll play with intensity. I am a very competitive person, and like to win. Even though I am not that great at basketball, when I participated in a league last year, I hustled like my life depended on it. Because I wanted to win, it was pretty easy to get intense.

- Use music, which I mentioned in an earlier chapter. Allowing yourself to get into the emotion of a song can really ramp up your intensity.

- Find an exercise you enjoy. Find something you personally enjoy and do it. Something you are good at and enjoy will get you more excited and make you more likely to exercise with intensity.

- Mentally prepare yourself. Remind yourself why you are at the gym and that the temporary difficulty is worth it in the end.

Remember, this tip is not about overdoing it. It's about reaching an intensity level high enough to achieve benefits from a workout. You never want to overdo any activity to the point of health danger or injury.

Today ramp up your exercise intensity a little.

- Jonathan

CHAPTER 32

DO WHATEVER YOU CAN TO EXERCISE

Let's face it. Getting motivated to exercise is probably the biggest obstacle to actually exercising. It isn't easy to get up at 5:00 AM and hit the gym before work, or go for a run at 5:00 PM after a long day at work.

I once overheard an older gentleman at the YMCA talking to his friend who had not been to the gym recently. He told his friend that he had never left the gym feeling worse than when he entered, and in fact most times left feeling much better. I thought about it and totally agree.

With the exception of the odd days where I may have slightly injured myself or was sick, I always left the YMCA feeling better. I always had more energy (in spite of sometimes hour long workouts), better mental clarity, and greater self-esteem.

The same is true of when I run. I often start a run dragging. There are some days when the first mile is literally more challenging than the tenth mile. Yet, after a few miles, almost without fail, I always "settle in" and start feeling great.

If only we had the energy and mental clarity to get motivated to exercise!

The key is to remind yourself how good you will feel when you are done, not only the temporary sense of well-being, but also the great feeling you have being fit and thin.

Here a few of my personal ways to get yourself to a gym, track, or wherever you exercise.

- Just go. No matter how you feel, get in the car or get changed into your exercise clothes. Even if you have a million excuses, just get in your car, get in the gym, and get changed. You'll feel pretty silly if you back out at that point. Sometimes just being there is a good motivator.

- Visualize and feel the outcome. Visualize a timeline in front of you, going left to right, with the past to your left, the present at a point in front of you, and the future to your right. Visualize yourself feeling great after a workout on the right side of the timeline. Really feel how great you'll feel after an amazing workout.

Now, visualize that "feeling good" version of you moving from the future side of the timeline to the present of the timeline, right in front of you. Then, take a step forward and "step into" the "feeling good" version of yourself. Now, feel good in the present and get motivated!

- Recognize and avoid your distractions. I always go to the gym after work. If I go home, get on the couch or the computer and start my evening business, I am stuck. The motivation is gone. After work, I may be a little tired, but in the car I'm in the gym zone.

- Get a little help. Have a cup of coffee or tea beforehand if you're low on energy. Most of us are busy people and the gym is a lot of effort. Sometimes we need a little boost. Avoid a lot of caffeine, though, as it can be counterproductive because it can dehydrate you or make you jumpy.

- Keep a symbol of your goal. Keep a "fat picture" around or something along those lines with you at all times. Then, when you're ready to make excuses remind yourself how much you prefer being thin and fit.

Remember to use these tricks when you suddenly find yourself low on energy or making excuses why you can't exercise.

Today, if you "just aren't feeling" exercising, use one of the techniques above to get motivated!

- Jonathan

CHAPTER 33

DO IT YOURSELF

When most people think of exercise, they think of joining a gym, riding a bicycle, playing a sport, or going for a long run. Sure, these are all examples of exercise, but many people aren't very motivated to exercise because they may not like doing any of those things.

Fortunately, exercise is simply movement and physical exertion. Thus, virtually any activity can count as exercise. There are many types of activities that we frequently automate or pay someone else to do that burn a lot of calories. This could include doing yardwork or housework.

My personal example came in the winter of 2008 when I bought a new house and had to deal with the issue of snow (I lived in the Ohio Snowbelt) on my driveway. Paying someone to plow my driveway would cost around 500 dollars; I could do it for free.

I discovered that shoveling the driveway was not only cost effective, but also darn good exercise! In fact, snow shoveling burns around seven calories a minute and judging by my soreness the next day, also works the muscles pretty nicely!

Another suggestion may be to mow the yard with a push mower instead of a riding mower. And, in these times of economic uncertainty, it makes sense, if a person is healthy and able-bodied, to find ways to take on a few more activities that also burn calories.

Here are a few of my personal favorites:

- Shovel your walk or driveway.

- Walk to the post office.

- Mow the lawn with a push mower.

- Hand wash an article of clothing.

- Build something.

- Dig something (although it better be needed or your spouse may get annoyed).

- Wash your windows.

- Clean your gutters.

- Trip the hedges (even with an electric trimmer this is work!).

While some of these may not be adequate as your main intense exercise activity for the day, all of these burn extra calories.

Today find something that needs done which requires physical activity, and get to work!

- Jonathan

CHAPTER 34

KEEP IT OUT OF THE HOUSE

Most people wouldn't expect an alcoholic to have much success if she worked as a bartender, or a guy trying to be celibate visiting strip clubs. Yet, this is what those of us who eat too much often do when we keep foods in the house that lead us to temptation.

I know what foods trigger binge eating for me: cheese curls, fudge, snickers bars, and pretty much any snack food. The problem with a lot of these foods is that it is hard for me to just eat one serving. I want to eat more and more.

In order for me to maintain a healthy weight, I know that for me, I have to simply keep them out of the house. Any other solution will usually result in me eating way too many of them.

So, the solution is to keep them out of the house. Don't buy them.

But, what if someone *gives* them to you? I have a very simple solution. Give them to somebody else. One of David's students always brings him Skittles, because he likes them so much (they are, by the way, a food he loves, but has to avoid). While the temptation is to eat the entire bag, instead he shares them with the class. When friends and relatives get him snacks or candy, he spreads the love to his students.

Keeping food "out of the house" can be difficult when you live with other people who may not share your values, or, to be fair, your food addiction. This can be especially difficult if you have a family.

In some cases, I've had to put my foot down for the sake of health within my own family. For example, I don't allow deep fried snacks in the house except occasionally. Nor do I allow pop or sugary drinks. However, I can't expect my family to embrace all my choices, especially since not everyone has a problem with food. There has to be some compromise.

It may sound weird, but if you have someone in your house who insists on bringing food in that causes you problems, ask them to hide it. It sounds juvenile, but the phrase "out of sight, out of mind" holds true.

If I see a candy bar sitting around tempting me, I'm more likely to eat it than if I have to search the entire house for it.

Basically, my general advice is if you don't want to eat it, then don't buy it or have it around you. Conversely, if you think you should be eating it, buy it. Then when you're hungry and go to grab something, healthy will be your only option.

Today look at all the foods in your house that tempt you. Make sure they aren't on your list the next time you shop!

- Jonathan

CHAPTER 35

BREAK COMMON FOOD CONVENTIONS

When I was making lunch a few days ago I couldn't find a side dish for my low carb wrap. This wrap consists of turkey lunchmeat, a low carb tortilla, light mayonnaise, and mixed salad greens to create a wrap that tastes great and fills me up. I really do like it.

The problem was that I couldn't find a side dish to go with it. Usually, I will bring pistachios, peanuts, or if I have some as leftovers, something like cabbage and (whole wheat, low-carb) noodles. That morning I was stuck.

That got me thinking of something that has helped me lose weight over the years: challenging and then defying traditional conventions about food. I asked myself, "*Why did I need a side dish at all?*"

So, I decided to just make a second wrap instead of trying to find a side dish. Why? Because not only would it be healthier, but it was actually what I wanted to eat.

My grandma is the queen of food conventions, so I'll list a few things I have heard her say over the years. Some of them include:

- Every meal has to end with a dessert.

- You can't drink coffee after the morning.

- Eggs are only for breakfast.

- Sandwiches must have a bun.

- You have to eat three meals a day.

- Every meal should have a side dish.

- You have to drink milk to have strong bones.

- Mashed potatoes go with steak.

- You can't eat the same meal twice in a week.

- Kale juice? That's just weird.

- Spicy foods aggravate your digestive system.

- You must have rolls or biscuits with a meal.

- You should stuff yourself during the holidays. That's what people do!

You get the point. The problem with these "conventions" is that they can all be used to make you eat things that go against your healthy lifestyle choices. Below I list convention-defying responses to each of the ones listed above. Hopefully you can see how breaking them, and thinking outside of the box, can actually improve your health. I'm sure you have your own conventions you feel the need to follow, so be sure to challenge your own conventions too.

- Meals can end anyway you want them to. Heck, I recently ended a grilled chicken wrap meal with a turkey hot dog. How's that for "dessert?" I'll save the extra calories and sugar and end the meal without dessert, or with something else.

- I'll drink coffee in the afternoon and evening if I want, because not only does coffee have a variety of health benefits, but drinking it helps me avoid overeating.

- Eggs are a cheap, low carb, and filling food that taste good all day.

- A sandwich wrapped in lettuce saves me anywhere from 120-300 calories and lots of carbs. I'll choose that over bread I barely appreciate.

- I can eat as many meals a day as I feel is healthy. Some days I eat a large dinner and I'm just not hungry at breakfast. I have no need to eat and consume extra calories if I'm not hungry.

- Why does a meal have to have what is traditionally classified as a "side dish?" A great low carb and high protein meal for me would be steak with a side of chicken breast.

- There are a variety of ways to get calcium and other minerals besides milk.

- I prefer asparagus, green beans, or broccoli with my steak, and those save me a lot of calories and carbs.

- If I eat the same healthy and good tasting meal multiple times a week – or even multiple times a day – what does it matter?

- I personally take pride in eating healthy food, whether it is "weird" or not.

- Actually, spicy foods may make my digestive system even healthier, and possibly boost my metabolism.

- Meals can taste just as good without extra bread (and the calories and carbs that go with it).

- You can eat healthily and stick to your eating plan on any day of the year.

In conclusion, challenging cultural conventions and expectations about food can help you make healthy choices.

Today identify some cultural food conventions that keep you unhealthy. What one can you break today?

- David

CHAPTER 36

SUPPLEMENTS

I've been into vitamins and other supplements for years, but I had fallen into a habit of taking them only occasionally, which given my poor diet (I literally ate sausage pasta for dinner every night for several months), meant that I was probably not reaching optimal levels of certain nutrients if not being outright deficient!

That changed on August 6th in 2007 when I decided to get serious about my health. Other than purposefully taken "vitamin holidays" I've always taken my supplements. And, I've noticed positive differences in my general health from them.

For example, in spite of vigorous workouts 6-7 days a week, I never have experienced joint pain. I attribute that, in addition to having strong quadriceps muscles, to taking Glucosamine Sulfate, Chondroitin, and MSM.

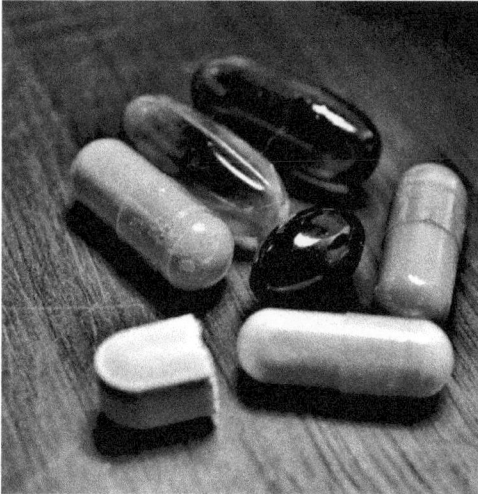

If I need a little mental boost, especially before workouts, I take an Acetyl L-Carnitine or DMAE pill. I take Green Tea to help my metabolism and for a little caffeine boost, also at the beginning of workouts. I also take proteolytic enzymes on an empty stomach before workouts, because studies have shown a preventative anti-inflammatory effect (24).

Are there any proven supplements that help with weight loss? Probably some. David wrote in a previous chapter about emerging research on betaine.

However, in most cases, don't believe the hype about weight loss supplements. In fact, disbelieve most of it.

Most of the formulas you see in health magazines probably do little or nothing to actually aid weight loss. Most may just be energy boosters and you can get that from better sources and more cheaply.

And, *no* supplement is a magic bullet to cause weight loss without proper eating and exercise. I do, however, believe that certain supplements can *help* with weight loss and issues associated with it.

Caffeine from green tea could give you more energy and some studies have shown a metabolic benefit (25). A small study suggested Vitamins B12 and B6 might help overweight people lose weight (26). Chromium supplementation has been shown to possibly reduce carbohydrate cravings (27). Vitamin D may have a role in weight loss too (28).

Other energy/mood boosting supplements are Acetyl L-Carnitine, Beta-Alanine, and DMAE.

Fish Oil and Glucosamine Sulfate, along with proteolytic enzymes such as Bromelain, seem to help moderate joint problems.

I would recommend researching supplements very carefully and then making a decision about which ones to take with your doctor. Also, shop around. One a recent trip, I noticed a gas station was selling a single pill for seven dollars. It was packaged to look like it was some sort of magic weight loss enhancer. I looked at the ingredients and they were herbs, vitamins, and minerals that I could have purchased for about five cents a pill. So, if you must buy a weight loss supplement, at least pay a fair price.

Today check out your supplements. Don't expect any magic, but are you getting the weight loss supplements you need?

- Jonathan

CHAPTER 37

THE MOST IMPORTANT MEAL OF THE DAY

David already mentioned that eating eggs or another high protein food for breakfast provides a weight loss advantage that lasts throughout the whole day. However, what about eating breakfast itself? Is that a way to lose weight?

Yes, it seems that mom and our kindergarten teachers were right on this one. A recent study showed, for example, that teens who ate breakfast were on average five pounds skinnier than those who skipped breakfast, in spite of the breakfast eaters consuming more total daily calories. I have my theories about why this is the case (29).

My main one is that eating earlier helps you feel full later. Your body has its need for food satisfied, as opposed to being forced to wait for food later. All of us know the feeling of starvation we get when we wait forever to eat. Eating breakfast satisfies those hunger signals and keeps them more level throughout the day.

I can see why people would want to skip breakfast; I used to do it all the time. I'd say "coffee was enough" or "I didn't have time." Plus, many times in the morning, we just don't feel like eating.

And, many of us associate breakfast with bacon, doughnuts, and other pretty unhealthy items. However, we can't survive on coffee (even if I wish we could). It's important to eat something even if it's small, and breakfast can and should be healthy.

I typically eat light yogurt, fruit, oatmeal, or eggs. If you take a multi-vitamin in the morning, make sure to include a little fat to help some of the vitamins absorb.

However, you still have to watch your calorie intake at breakfast. Eating too much not only increases your daily total calories, but a huge breakfast can make you sluggish the rest of the morning. If you follow the rest of the tips in this book, your breakfast can make your day even more healthy!

Today give breakfast a try, if you normally don't. Try some eggs for an added weight loss advantage.

- Jonathan

CHAPTER 38

KNOW HOW TO HANDLE THE HOLIDAYS

The word holiday comes from the combination of the words holy and day which is appropriate since most of our holidays are holy in the true sense of the word (e.g. Christmas and Easter) or hallowed in a broad sense (e.g. Independence Day and Veterans Day). In addition, holidays are typically times of happiness, family, and festivity. However, for people trying to lose weight or maintain a healthy eating and fitness plan, the holidays can seem a little less wonderful.

We've all been there: the seemingly endless food, the constant lounging, and perhaps worst of all, the

silent peer pressure to engage in it all (or maybe this
is just my family!).

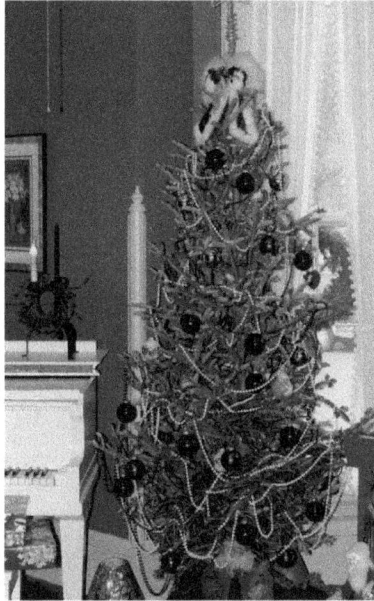

I think one of the primary reasons the holidays
are often so stressful to dieters or those trying to
remain healthy and fit is that the regular schedules
and habits we try to develop are often severely
disrupted. So, the challenge of the dieter or the person
trying to maintain healthy habits is to find a way to
keep up the healthy habits throughout the holidays
(yes, even one day often gets stretched to days, or in
the case of Christmas, weeks).

It's not always easy since, for many, holidays involve staying in other people's homes, eating other people's cooking, and even if we are the ones in charge, we still have to deal with other people's expectations which are often quite stringent (try serving fruit instead of pie at Thanksgiving and see what happens!).

So, how can you keep to your healthy eating and fitness habits? Here are a few tips, but they assume you have the habits to begin with!

1. Keep your own schedule intact. I believe that keeping your routine relatively unchanged is vital to survive the holidays. If you eat yogurt and a banana for breakfast and go to the gym at 11:30 AM during most weeks, try to keep up those habits during the holidays too. Not possible? See #2.

2. Be flexible with the times, but not the content. Okay, maybe Grandma Ethel insists that everyone gather for a family photo at 11:30 AM. That's fine. Then, plan on going to the gym at noon. Family boggle game at noon? Then absolutely insist on 1:00 PM. Be flexible with the times, but if you go to the gym every other day during your normal life, keep to this during the holidays.

3. Be firm. If you interact with family members during the holidays, chances are many will not share your health and fitness vision. Fine, and you should respect that.

But, they must respect you too. If Grandma Ethel insists on a family photo and boggle, then you can also insist on a healthy addition to the family meal and time for a walk. Give and take, but don't just give, give, give and gain five pounds.

4. Find allies. Maybe cousin Bernice is also into health and fitness. Team up with her and work together, whether it's to fight temptation or go to the gym.

5. Don't expect others to do it. In most cases, your family isn't out to sabotage your efforts. They may either not care about health personally or not know how important it is to you.

Don't assume the worst, but also don't assume others will do your work for you. If you want tofu turkey, don't insist that Uncle Gino make it in place of his usual turkey. Let Uncle Gino do his thing and you make tofu turkey too. People may think you're weird, but they won't think you're a complainer who expects everyone to hand you everything.

6. Adapt, adapt, and adapt. I know I said to keep your schedule first and then be flexible about time only. Now, I'm giving more contradictory advice. See this as a "plan C" option.

If you can't keep your normal schedule, be flexible about the times. If you can't keep to your normal content, then adapt. For example, if you travel to see family and they don't have a gym that allows visitors nearby, then run or walk.

If it's the middle of winter, then jog in place. Boring? Sure. But, it's better than nothing and it's only for a couple of days. If your family only offers high calorie foods at dinner and you haven't cooked anything, then just eat small portions, even if you're used to eating bigger portions of healthier food.

7. Pick your battles. No one likes a whiner and getting labeled a health or fitness freak will just make others tune out your views. So, choose your battles carefully. Decide which issues you will compromise on and which you will fight (politely) for. Be willing to accommodate as much as possible, but stick to your guns on essentials.

For example, if you don't eat red meat as a matter of conviction, then don't eat it, even if Aunt Gertrude insists it puts meat on your bones (whey protein powder is fine, thanks). On the other hand, if you prefer running in the mornings, don't skip church with the family on Easter when you can just as easily run in the afternoon. The former makes you look principled; the latter just petty.

8. Indulge a little. Have a piece of pie; enjoy the extra cup of coffee; eat grandma's stuffing. You may not normally do some of these things, but these are holidays.

Enjoy the more decadent foods in moderation or small amounts occasionally and you'll be less likely to binge later. The holidays are a great time to let yourself indulge a little. Emphasis on a little, not indulge. Repeat that as a mantra.

9. Finally, enjoy the holidays. Holidays are supposed to be fun and too much strategizing about health and fitness could ruin that. Then again, so could gaining ten pounds from Thanksgiving to New Year's.

So, plan ahead, follow this advice, and it should make your holiday more fun, less stressful, and most importantly, from a health and fitness perspective, less likely to result in those jeans feeling a good deal tighter.

Today think about your next holiday dinner and how you will stick to your health plan.

- Jonathan

CHAPTER 39

GET LOADED WITHOUT LOADING UP ON CALORIES

I have a friend on Facebook who is always complaining about her inability to lose weight. If you hear her talk about it, losing weight is next to impossible. She claims she's tried everything, but just can't do it! Then, you look in her pictures and you see that she drinks alcohol...a lot.

If you want to lose weight and like to drink, keep it under control or you'll be adding hundreds of pointless calories to your diet weekly (maybe daily). Your average non-light beer has around 150 calories. A glass of wine has around 130. A shot of liquor 80. Cocktails are the worst, with sangria coming in at 225 and a Piña Colada at 340!

And, while some people drink in moderation, many drink to excess, even if it's only a few times a month. But, even moderate drinking of wine might add as many as 600 calories a week. A Saturday night bender on mixed drinks could set someone back around 1500 calories. Those numbers can really start to add up. And, those translate into pounds.

In addition, alcohol actually makes you hungrier. So, if you go out and drink (even to the point of "just buzzing") you'll likely be tempted to eat, especially junk. This happens for a few reasons.

First, alcohol calories are empty. Like sugary drinks, they "count" as calories (possibly), but they don't satisfy hunger. So, you can consume 300 calories of beer but your body doesn't see it as getting you any more full. So, you still have the urge to eat.

Second, alcohol loosens inhibitions. So, just like a person might put a lampshade on his head and have sex with a random stranger under the influence, the mental discipline to stay on a diet and not eat that plate of bacon cheese fries also disappears...and eventually the cheese fries disappear too.

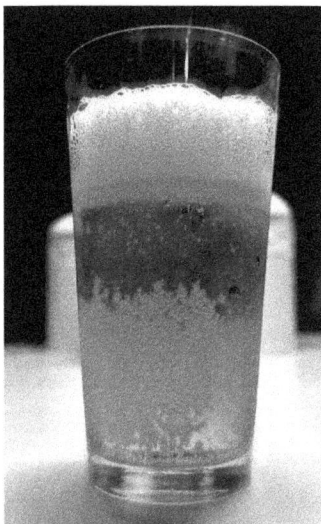

Finally, alcohol stimulates the hypothalamus, the part of the brain that regulates sleep, body temperature, and hunger. When it gets triggered, you are tempted to eat when you normally wouldn't want to eat. So, that's why when you get drunk you may put away a whole pizza and wake up regretting it.

So, as you can see, drinking alcohol can really sabotage a diet if you're not careful. If you enjoy drinking, especially a lot, you will definitely need to cut back if you want to lose weight. We have a word for a guy who drinks a six pack of beer every night and it's not just alcoholic. It's fat. But, if you like to drink, here a few tips to do it and still lose or maintain your weight.

First, choose the lightest options possible. For example, drink light beer, dry wines, or mixed drinks with diet components (like vodka and diet tonic or fruity drinks with sugar free syrups). This option could save you hundreds of calories.

Just keep in mind, these drinks don't typically have less alcohol, so don't be irresponsible and think you can drink more.

Second, don't drink on an empty stomach. Eat something healthy either before you drink or while you are drinking. This will slow down the alcohol absorption, which ideally would mean that you drink less. It also means that your body will signal that you are full and you're less likely to binge eat later.

Third, keep your drinking moderate, even when you "go out." If you only have two or three over several hours, you'll not only keep your composure, you'll also not risk doing anything stupid (especially driving). In addition, you'll save hundreds of calories over your friend who is having nine or ten.

Finally, perhaps the best thing you can do regarding drinking is just to not do it, especially if you find yourself losing control or the tendency towards alcoholism runs in your family. Alcohol only temporarily solves problems and usually creates worse ones down the line (maybe even the next day). And, if you drink a lot often, then your weight loss goals will take a lot longer to reach.

Detoxing from alcohol if you drink a lot can be fatal. So, if you decide to give it up completely and you are a heavy drinker, definitely consult your doctor. He can hook you up with detox and a treatment program.

Technically, a gram of alcohol has seven calories, making it more calorie dense than carbs or proteins. However, some research indicates the body doesn't utilize alcohol calories as energy the same way it does other calories (especially the more you drink in a smaller time frame), and therefore alcohol doesn't have the weight gaining effect of other calories. There is still a lot of debate about what happens to alcohol calories, so don't assume that alcohol "doesn't count."

Today evaluate your alcohol consumption and ask where you can and should cut back.

- Jonathan

CHAPTER 40

GETTING OVER SEASONAL PITFALLS

As I was thinking about weight loss yesterday, I realized that I often notice seasonal patterns in my weight gain and weight loss. It is difficult to notice overarching seasonal patterns, because I have been fat in all seasons, and thin in all seasons, but there are a few observable patterns. Below, I share some of my observations related to each season.

I am using this chapter as a chance to also share some of the more personal aspects of my weight loss journey. I hope that they can help you identify your patterns and confront some of your seasonal issues.

<u>Spring</u>

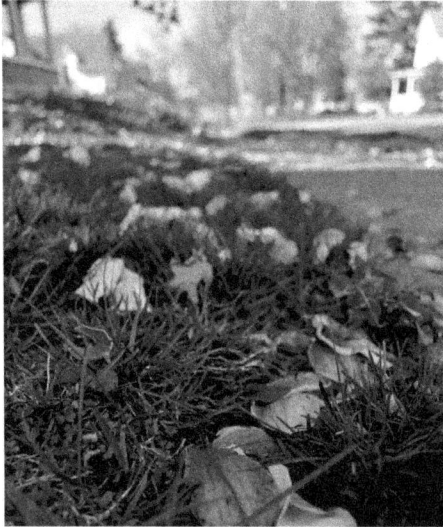

I have memories of gaining weight in the spring. The reason is simple: I often am successful in losing weight in the winter, and by spring, I become complacent. Common sense dictates that I should actually lose weight in the spring: the weather is getting nicer, and my body is getting out of hibernation mode. However, spring brings complacency for me, and while I am not sure why, I always seem to get really hungry in the spring.

Spring weight gain started in high school. I remember lifting weights a lot my sophomore year in the fall and winter, yet I regularly skipped weight lifting in the spring to hang out with girls. I gained about fifteen pounds that spring because I spent most of the time sitting on my butt. My junior year in high school was different, when I started training for a 100 mile bike ride. I spent many nights and weekends riding that bike, and got in great shape!

Nonetheless, spring has more often than not brought complacency. Last year, tortilla chips were my weakness. Man, from March until May, I ate tons of them, with meals and as snacks, often with fresh salsa. I finally had to just get them out of the house, and I rarely buy them to this day! When I go out to eat, I still put them away...but that is another post.

For example, one spring in particular I had various weaknesses, mainly eating too many meals out because of the special events I was involved in: prom, the school auction, the New York City trip, honor society induction, spring break, National Speaker Association meetings, dinner with the visiting retreat team tonight at school, etc.

It seems like there were so many special occasions that spring, and so many occasions for eating too much! It was also harder to exercise regularly when my evenings were busy. I should have been able to have dealt with that, and I did by saving calories certain places, and by exercising more, but that spring was a real battle.

Below is my special plan to avoid weight gain in the spring:

- Avoid eating too much (since my appetite seems to grow in the spring).

- Get out on the days I can. I love running outside, and since it rains a lot in the spring, getting out often requires some planning.

- Connect to the symbol of spring as a time of renewal, and use it to "spring clean" my health.

Summer

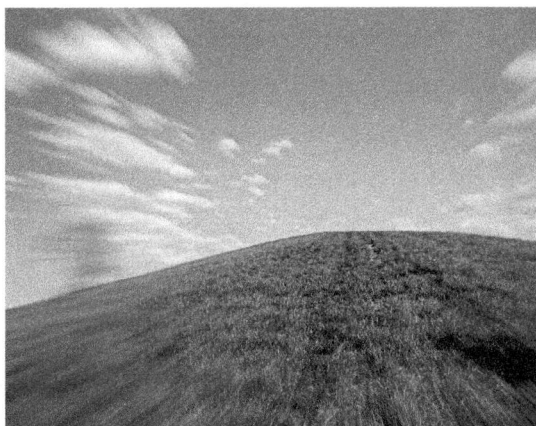

I have great memories of recent summers, but in high school, it was hardly my favorite season. Why would I not like a sunny, three month break from school? In a word, football. I enjoyed football, but it was very tough, and required a lot of commitment.

We began weight-lifting and running in June, practicing in July, and we began full practices (including "two-a-days" from 7:30 AM - 3:30 PM) by August. Hence, I basically had no summer "break." Football got me in shape that is for sure, but because it was stressful on my body and mind, I tended to compensate by eating.

After a seven hour practice, nothing satisfied like a huge, greasy, meal of two ham-and-cheese subs, French fries, and loads of pop. For this reason, I rarely began diets or health programs in the summer during high school. The only exception is the summer before my junior year, when I continued an exercise program I began with spring bike riding. I exercised diligently with my brother Jonathan, and friend, Mike.

We lifted every other day, and ran outside at the school track afterward. By the end of July, I worked my way up to running six miles. I continued running on Sundays (my football off-day) once school had started. I still look back fondly on those Sunday runs,

not to date as much, or even concern myself with dating, during the season.

After football, I was ready to re-enter the social scene, and I knew then, as I know now, that being fit provides a social advantages, so I took my weight loss seriously. It is a shame that just as my diets were beginning, Thanksgiving and Christmas were coming up. It was bad timing on my part, but I managed.

In high school, I recall going to the Y a lot during the fall, and it was during the tail end of the autumn that I usually resumed weight-lifting. Since graduating from all schooling, the fall doesn't have the social significance it once did, so I haven't begun many health programs in the fall lately, but I typically do pretty well at continuing them in the fall. Halloween, Thanksgiving, and December festivities provide some temptations, but there are strategies to help me avoid putting on the pounds during holidays.

To lose weight in the fall, I need to remember to:

- Keep my Halloween, Thanksgiving, and December eating under control.

- Make good use of the sunny, warm, fall days, when I can get out and run.

- Get out and hike and/or walk on days when it may be too cold to run, but perfect for bundling up and hiking.

Winter

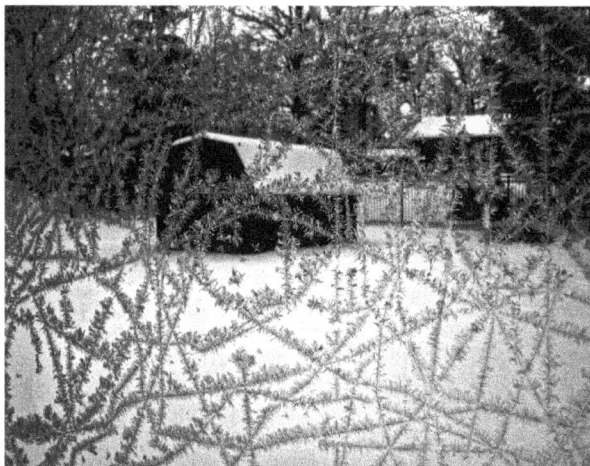

Winter is a rough time for me all around. As I get older, I dislike winter more and more. Growing up, winter was almost magical: Christmas (and all associated content, including lights), snow days, warm fires, and so forth, stoked my imagination. Even though this past winter was cold and dreary to a large degree, the "greeting card" winter of my nostalgia still shapes my view of winter.

These days, outside of Christmas, I can do without the winter. Seriously, the less winter, the better. I often joke that I wish the cold and snow would end at Christmas: I would like a cold and snowy Christmas, and by the middle of January, the days can warm up to the 60s as far as I'm concerned. Let me say that I can appreciate the winter on certain levels, and I will always love the "four seasons," but winter is just too limiting.

In high school, I usually lost weight in the winter, not because winter provides any kind of advantage (it actually may provide a disadvantage to weight loss because it drives our body into a kind of "hibernation"), but because, as I've mentioned, winter is when my social life, which began in the fall, was revving up. I had already begun losing weight in the fall, and this continued, and even increased, in the winter. This, and the new year, provided a strong motivation to get the Y, and eat right.

These days, winter doesn't cause me too many weight-related problems. I sometimes struggle with infections and mild mood issues, but this doesn't directly relate to my weight. During winter, my main issue is that I have to make my exercise interesting. This is always the struggle for me in the winter. Usually, there is one effective solution to this problem: music. In high school, I had a cassette

Walkman. I discovered "oldies" during this time, so I would make mix tapes of oldies I got off the radio and various CDs, non-creatively titled "The Exercise Collection" 1-2. I upgraded to a Discman around 2000, and in 2008, I finally got a MP3 player. Right now, I am listening to Avicii, which is upbeat enough to make exercise easier. Basically, to lose weight in the winter I need to:

- Make effective use of music, to keep exercise interesting.

- Vary my exercise routine enough to keep interested.

- Not let winter blahs negatively affect my weight loss.

- Get out on the few good days that the winter offers.

Today identify any seasonal pitfalls that may be stopping you from sticking to your health goals, and rectify them.

- David

FREQUENTLY ASKED QUESTIONS

1. Do you have a diet you recommend?

We are not dieticians, so we cannot recommend a specific diet. Generally, a diet that restricts calories will cause weight loss. However, we find that specific food choices can improve personal well-being and speed up weight loss.

Personally, Jonathan and I prefer a "lower carb" diet, that is also relatively low in calories (1700-2200 per day). We both try to avoid refined grain products (those made of white flour or white sugar), and generally keep our "net carbs" in a 75-175 gram range. We don't make much of an attempt to restrict fat. We also eat generous amounts of fruits, vegetables, and high fiber/low-carb products. We also eat a lot fish.

I flirted with a low fat diet back in the 1990s. I always felt hungry, was tired in the afternoon, and gained weight back quickly. Since switching to a lower carb diet I have a lot fewer cravings and feel much more mentally stable.

2. What kind of exercises do you do?

We both run a lot in the warmer months. In the winter, we will attempt to run, unless snow gets in the way. We also regularly do workout programs like Insanity and Asylum. For fun we run "extreme races" like the Tough Mudder and Warrior Dash. However, there are a lot of options available, so do whatever you find interesting and be open to finding newer and exciting options to prevent boredom.

3. I have tried to lose weight in the past. Why will your tips help me actually lose it this time?

As we mentioned in certain chapters, most people are prone to underestimating their caloric intake in a given day. They are also bad at knowing how many calories are in a food, unless they look it up. Our tips encourage accuracy and honesty with yourself. Also, most people don't have a full "arsenal" of weight loss tools at their disposal. In this book we have given you forty new weapons in your weight loss arsenal. Even if you implement a few of them, you'll find that you'll likely lose some weight.

4. I'm not seeing results. What am I doing wrong?

Your body loves homoeostasis, i.e. equilibrium. It resists change. Every time I have attempted to lose weight, it took me a few months to see any significant results. I attribute this to the former point, homeostasis, but also to the fact that if you are attempting to lose weight the right way, by including exercise, you are also likely gaining muscle in addition to losing fat. So, you may lose a pound of fat, but may have gained a pound of muscle as well. I suggest gauging your initial success on how you look and feel until your weight catches up.

-David

The Basic Math Of Losing Weight

Determining why you may or may not be losing weight is complicated because of metabolism issues, muscle gain/loss, and other variables, but in the end, weight loss and gain are the result of basic math. My goal in this brief essay is to get you to think about the role of calorie counting in weight loss, and provide you with some tools to effectively gauge your daily calorie needs.

While the real situation is more complex, a good rule of thumb is that basically, 3500 calories is equivalent to one pound of body fat. Thus, to lose a pound of body fat, you must burn 3500 more calories than you eat over a given period of time (30, 31).

Let's say one day of the week you labor during the day and go to the Y in the evening. On this day, you burn a massive 4500 calories. However, because you have no time to eat this day, you only consume 1000 calories. In this scenario, you would lose a pound of body fat, at least theoretically.

Now, let's apply this math to weight gain. Let's say you pig out at the all-you-can-eat buffet, and after the sixth plate, you have consumed 5200 calories that day (this is high, but not impossible for people who go overboard at a buffet). And, you worked all day taking calls in a cubicle, so you burned only 1700 calories. You have, in theory, just gained a pound of fat. As this example shows, in modern America, it is far easier to gain an excess 3500 calories, than to burn them, as this scenario is more plausible than the first example.

This is where Fitday, My Fitness Pal, or other calorie-tracking programs are helpful. Personally, I use Fitday, so that will be my example. They are all very similar. Fitday has a cool feature that allows you to program in a weight loss goal, and the date for that goal. Then, it calculates how many pounds a week you have to lose to reach that goal. And here comes the really cool part...Fitday also calculates how many calories you must restrict each day to meet your goal (using the 3500 number I have mentioned).

My goal, when I originally wrote this essay, was to lose thirteen pounds by Labor Day. To do this, I had to burn 875 more calories per day than I consumed. Obviously, weight loss was not this simple for me, because of other variables like my muscle gain from weight lifting, but nonetheless, I find this a very helpful tool for gauging how well I do on a particular day. This allows me to eat a little more on days when I exercise a lot, because the goal is based on calorie restriction, not on a set number of calories per day.

Using one magic calorie number for every single day is too static, artificial, and unhelpful, because some days we are going to burn more calories than others. Consuming a few extra calories on these active days may not hurt our goal, and even help us by keeping us satisfied. Below are some images of what I am talking about.

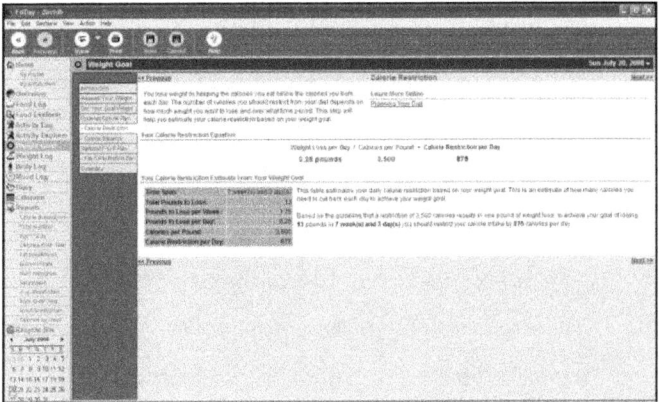

In the above image, I am on "step 5" of the Fitday weight assessment process, in which I have planned the calorie restriction needed to lose my desired weight. Fitday software does the math for me, based on what I set as my weight goals in an earlier step.

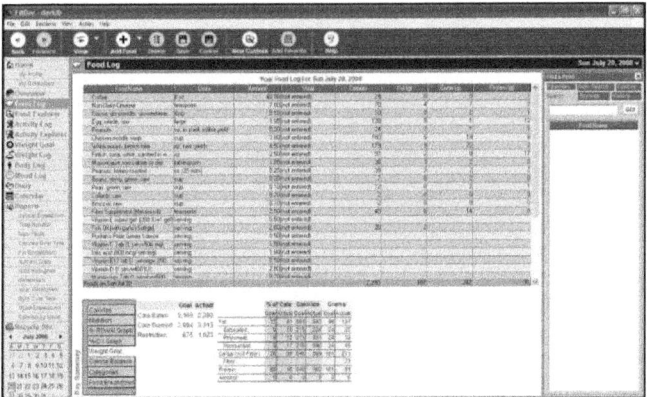

In the second image, above, I have consumed more calories than Fitday estimates I need to consume to meet my weight goal. However, there are no worries for this day, because I am active: in the end, I have burned 1023 more calories than I consumed, which is over the 875 I need to restrict to meet my weight goal on time.

If you don't want to bother downloading an app or software to determine how many calories you need to restrict to lose weight, check out the TDEE Calculator at http://www.iifym.com/tdee-calculator.

As you can see losing weight is about numbers: calories consumed, and calories burned. While there are other factors involved, recognizing the importance of calories, and keeping track of your calorie consumption and expenditure, will aid you in whatever weight loss efforts you undertake.

Before I end this article, I want to mention something about metabolism. As Dr. Mark Hyman points out in his book *Ultrametabolism*, all calories are not necessarily equal when it comes to gaining or losing weight (32).

For example, 100 calories from a Coke or Pepsi is going to have a more disastrous effect on your weight than 100 calories from kidney beans. The reason is that the 100 calories from cola are from high fructose corn syrup, which enters the blood stream immediately, so the calories not immediately utilized are stored as fat.

The 100 calories in kidney beans are absorbed more slowly because of the fiber in the beans, so they are absorbed and utilized over an extended period of time, which means they are more likely to be burned by the body, and less likely to be stored as fat. It is important to keep this in mind when choosing foods.

- David

SOURCES

REFERENCES

1.

psychology.about.com/od/socialpsychology/f/halo-effect.htm

2.

medicalnewstoday.com/articles/242089.php

3.

news.bbc.co.uk/2/hi/health/4211789.stm

4.

spineuniverse.com/wellness/exercise/build-muscle-lose-fat

5.

sciencedaily.com/releases/2008/02/080205161231.htm

6.

Larimore, Walter L., Sherri Flynt, and Steve Halliday.
    Super-Sized Kids: How to Rescue Your Child
    from the Obesity Threat. New York: Center
    Street, 2005.

7.

livescience.com/health/060703_sleep_less.html

8.

lifeinyouryears.net/blog/2008/10/26/artificial-light-at-
    night-raise-breast-cancer-risk/

9.

Cooper, Robert K., and Leslie Cooper. Flip The
    Switch: Proven Strategies To Fuel Your
    Metabolism & Burn Fat 24 Hours A Day.
    Emmaus, PA: Rodale, 2005.

10.

health.msn.com/fitness/abs/articlepage.aspx?cp-
    documentid=100204206

11.

mirror.co.uk/news/uk-news/pint-water-before-meals-
    secret-6324889

12.

ncbi.nlm.nih.gov/pubmed/1454084

13.

huffingtonpost.com/dr-mark-hyman/why-cholesterol-may-not-b_b_290687.html

14.

eurekalert.org/pub_releases/2008-08/epr-awe080408.php

15.

munews.missouri.edu/news-releases/2013/0326-protein-rich-breakfasts-prevent-unhealthy-snacking-in-the-evening-mu-researcher-finds

16.

livestrong.com/article/417287-how-do-monounsaturated-fats-help-you-to-lose-belly-fat/

17.

thepopularman.com/the-major-weight-loss-and-muscle-gain-supplement-nobody-knows-about-betaine/

18.

bodybuilding.com/fun/the-real-tabata-brutal-circuit-from-the-protocols-inventor.html

19.

thepopularman.com/what-is-tabata-and-why-you-should-use-it/

20.

umassmed.edu/news/news-archives/2015/02/when-it-comes-to-diets-one-simple-change-can-be-effective/

21.

ncbi.nlm.nih.gov/pubmed/1454084

22.

scientificamerican.com/article/psychology-workout-music/

23.

content.time.com/time/health/article/0,8599,1827342,00.html

24.

webmd.com/vitamins-and-supplements/lifestyle-guide-11/supplement-guide-bromelain-bromelin

25.

umm.edu/health/medical/altmed/herb/green-tea

26.

nutraingredients.com/Research/Chromium-B-vitamins-could-reduce-middle-aged-spread

27.

lifeinyouryears.net/blog/2008/10/06/chromium-picolinate-helps-you-eat-less/

28.

lifeinyouryears.net/blog/2009/02/21/vitamin-d-and-obesity/

29.

news.bbc.co.uk/2/hi/health/7275554.stm

30.

todaysdietitian.com/newarchives/111114p36.shtml

31.

mayoclinic.org/healthy-lifestyle/weight-loss/in-depth/calories/art-20048065

32.

Hyman, Mark. Ultrametabolism: The Simple Plan For Automatic Weight Loss. New York: Atria Books, 2008.

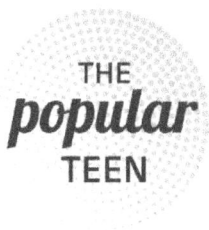

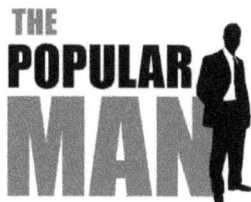

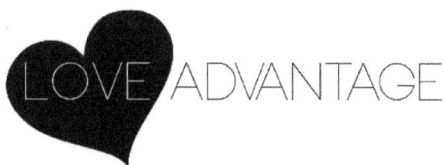

For more information on becoming your absolute best self, to become more confident, successful, and unstoppable, check out some of the authors' other websites. You can find plenty of FREE resources, and information about special events, classes, and consulting:

thepopularman.com
thepopularteen.com
loveadvantage.net

More Excellent Books

From Theta Hill Press And Our Partners:

thetahillpress.com

Be Popular Now: How Any Man Can Become Confident, Attractive and Successful (And Have Fun Doing It)

Any guy can develop the personality necessary to win friends, get dates, and have the career success he's dreamed of. This is the handbook of social success for guys. Any guy can learn the tips, tricks, and techniques necessary to transform from dull, boring, and dateless into a charming and fun guy whom everyone wants to get to know.

Eleven Dating Mistakes Guys Make (And How To Correct Them)

Many guys want dates, but can't seem to get them. The odds are good that if a guy is perpetually single, he is making most of these "dating mistakes." This is a no-nonsense guide to helping a guy get dates. This book tells the truth about attraction based on the science of human attraction.

Eleven Dating Mistakes Women Make (And How To Correct Them)

Some women have guys lined up to talk to them, while other women aren't as lucky. What do women who get dates do that single women don't? This book tells the truth about attraction. While many books sugar coat the issue, saying things like "be yourself and guys will like you," this book looks at the science of human attraction and explains the dating mistakes women often make.

The Teen Popularity Handbook: Make Friends, Get Dates, And Become Bully-Proof

Studies over and over again show the importance that social skills play in a person's social and career success. Most teens struggle with shyness and awkwardness, struggling to make friends, get dates, and stand up for themselves and others when necessary. This handbook provides tips and tricks to help any teen to become more popular, admired, and bully-proof, explained in a way teens can understand and implement. Parents are raving about the book too, because they know the importance personality plays in future career success.

Size Doesn't Matter: A Short Man's Handbook Of Dating And Relationship Success

It isn't easy being a short guy in the world of dating. Studies and polls show that women prefer taller guys, and short guys often find less success in their careers and relationships. This book provides short guys with all the tools necessary to attract the women of their dreams, and enter into positive relationships with them.

Say It Like You Mean It: How To Use Affirmations and Declarations To Create The Life You Want

Most of us have been exposed to years of negative thoughts, from both our own brains, and from other people. We have been conditioned to think in limiting ways. This is why we struggle to find success in life, and seem unable to achieve our health, career, and social goals, even though we desperately want to be successful. This book explains how to change your life, and rewire your brain, using the power of affirmations and declarations.